Mental Health Systems and Policy in Low- and Middle-Income Countries

Series Editor

S. M. Yasir Arafat, Bangladesh Specialized Hospital, Dhaka, Bangladesh

This series of books explores critical dimensions of mental health and psychology in low- and middle-income countries (LMICs), where the majority of people with mental illness live but access to care and research remains limited. Despite a significant disease burden, mental health services in LMICs face challenges such as inadequate infrastructure, workforce shortages, stigma, and high treatment gaps. These volumes aim to address these gaps by presenting culturally relevant, evidence-based insights and practical solutions tailored to resource-constrained settings.

Covering topics such as mental health services, epidemiology, social psychiatry, addiction, suicide prevention, psychiatric nursing, and the impact of climate change, migration, and disasters, the series integrates global perspectives with local realities. Each book emphasizes innovative interventions, policy recommendations, and strategies for improving mental health literacy and reducing stigma. Contributions from LMIC-based clinicians and researchers ensure authentic, context-specific knowledge.

Designed for academics, practitioners, policymakers, and students, this series provides a comprehensive platform for advancing research, informing practice, and supporting capacity building. By addressing underexplored areas and fostering inclusive discourse, it seeks to improve mental health outcomes and promote sustainable development across diverse LMIC settings.

S. M. Yasir Arafat · Hasina Akter
Editors

Psychiatric Nursing in Bangladesh

Springer

Editors
S. M. Yasir Arafat
Department of Psychiatry
Bangladesh Specialized Hospital
Dhaka, Bangladesh

Hasina Akter
Department of Graduate Nursing
Bangladesh Medical University
Dhaka, Bangladesh

ISSN 3120-4376 ISSN 3120-4384 (electronic)
Mental Health Systems and Policy in Low- and Middle-Income Countries
ISBN 978-981-95-8500-7 ISBN 978-981-95-8501-4 (eBook)
https://doi.org/10.1007/978-981-95-8501-4

This Springer imprint is published by the registered company Springer Nature Singapore Pte Ltd.
The registered company address is: 152 Beach Road, #21-01/04 Gateway East, Singapore 189721, Singapore

Preface

Bangladesh is a lower-middle-income densely populated South Asian country with around 170 million people facing a significant dual burden of communicable and non-communicable diseases. Non-communicable diseases make up about 60% of the health burden, with mental disorders among the top five, affecting 18.7% of the population. Despite bearing such a status, there is a critical shortage of mental health resources (human and financial) contributes to the treatment gap over 90%. There is an extreme shortage of mental health nurses in Bangladesh, as the latest estimate revealed that there are 0.43 psychiatric nurses for 100,000 population. There are about 80,000 registered nurses, and as per a cautious projection, the demand for nurses will be 483,000 in 2030. There are about 440 nursing institutes in Bangladesh; among them, BSc Nursing (4-year duration) has been offered in 192 institutes. Each year, approximately 35,000 nursing students enroll in programs across Bangladesh in the public and private sectors, yet they lack access to materials tailored to the unique challenges of psychiatric nursing within the country's cultural and healthcare context. Currently, no textbook is available in the country on psychiatric nursing, despite the country's need for psychiatric mental health education. This book, *Psychiatric Nursing in Bangladesh,* attempted to fill that important gap.

It contains 16 chapters as per the BSc Nursing Curriculum (2018) in Bangladesh. It follows the chapter contents as mentioned in the curriculum. The 1st chapter, *Introduction to Psychiatric Nursing*, includes the concept of psychiatric nursing and its importance, mental health, determinants of mental health, mental health illness continuum, determinants of mental illness, cultural and socioeconomic factors related to mental health care, ethical and legal issues, psychiatric nursing process, and community mental health nursing. The 2nd chapter, b*iopsychosocial theories of mental health and illness*, includes the biological model, social model, psychoanalytic model, interpersonal model, Lazarus's—theory of emotion, and crisis theory of mental illness and their perspectives for mental health nursing. The 3rd chapter, *psychotherapeutic modalities*, covers psychopharmacology and other biologic treatments, family interventions/ therapy, psychotherapy: individual and group, and psychiatric nursing interventions for mental disorders. The 4th chapter, *therapeutic communication and the therapeutic relationship*, includes therapeutic use of self, empathy, phases of the nurse-patient relationship, and therapeutic communication techniques for mental health nursing. The 5th chapter, *care of clients with schizophrenia and other psychotic disorders*, includes definition, etiology, signs and symptoms, cause, treatment, nursing problems, and interventions for psychotic disorders. The 6th chapter, care of clients with mood disorders, includes definition, etiology, signs and symptoms, cause, treatment, nursing problems, and interventions for mood disorders. The 7th chapter, *care of clients with anxiety disorders*, includes definition, etiology, signs and symptoms, cause, treatment, nursing problems, and interventions for persons with anxiety disorders. The 8th chapter, c*are of clients with psychosomatic illnesses and somatoform disorders*, includes definition, etiology, signs and symptoms, cause, treatment, nursing problems, and interventions for the disorders. The 9th chapter, c*are of clients with neuropsychiatric disorders: obsessive compulsive disorder*, includes definition, etiology, signs and symptoms, cause, treatment, nursing problems, and interventions for the disorders. The 10th chapter, c*are of clients with delirium dementia and other related disorders*, discusses the definition, etiology, signs and symptoms, cause, treatment, nursing problems, and interventions for persons with neuropsychiatric disorders. The 11th chapter, c*are of clients with substance-related disorders*, highlights definition, etiology, signs and symptoms, cause, treatment, nursing problems, and interventions for addictive disorders. The 12th chapter, c*are of clients with sexual disorders*, mentions definition, etiology, signs and symptoms, cause, treatment, nursing problems, and interventions for psychosexual dysfunctions. The next chapters discuss *care of clients with suicide: children,adolescents,adults and elders*, *emergency psychiatric nursing care,mental health promotion across the lifespan*, and *public and private systems of care for mental health,including referral system.* This book provides basic insights and culturally relevant skills to help bridge the health services in the country. Offering localized content, practical case studies, and context-specific interventions will equip the next generation of nurses to better serve the mental health needs of Bangladeshi communities.

There is no similar book in the market on psychiatric nursing in Bangladesh. Hence, this will be the first book of its kind according to the curriculum of BSc Nursing in Bangladesh. It highlights the evidence available in the local context of the Bangladesh. It will be a useful resource for policymakers and mental health services providers, academicians working on *Psychiatric Nursing in Bangladesh.*

Dhaka, Bangladesh S. M. Yasir Arafat
Dhaka, Bangladesh Hasina Akter

Contents

About the Editors

Dr. S. M. Yasir Arafat is currently working as an Associate Consultant of Psychiatry at Bangladesh Specialized Hospital, Dhaka, Bangladesh. He is an Associate Professor of Frontier University Garowe, Somalia, an Associate Fellow of the Bangladesh Academy of Sciences, and a Senior Research Fellow of the Biomedical Research Foundation, Bangladesh. He was affiliated with the University of Bristol, UK, as a Visiting Senior Research Associate (August 2021–2023) and an Honorary Research Fellow with Dnet (October 2023–25). He completed his MD in Psychiatry from Bangabandhu Sheikh Mujib Medical University, Dhaka, and his MBBS from the Dhaka Medical College, Bangladesh. He also did an MPH in Health Economics and an MBA in Marketing. Dr. Arafat has (co)authored more than 400 peer-reviewed articles and 50 book chapters, and (co)edited more than 15 books with Springer. He is the lead editor of the book series *South Asian Perspectives in Mental Health and Psychology* with Springer. He has been included in the global 2% researcher list in 2021–23, and 2025. He is an editorial member of more than 10 leading journals in mental health, published by Elsevier, Wiley, Springer, Routledge, and Sage. His research focused on mental health, suicidal behavior, psychometrics, panic buying, and psycho-sexual disorders.

Hasina Akter is currently working as an Assistant Professor of the Faculty of Nursing at Bangladesh Medical University, Dhaka, Bangladesh. She focuses on mental health and psychiatric nursing. She completed MSN in Mental Health & Psychiatric Nursing from the National Institute of Advanced Nursing Education and Research and BSc in Nursing from the Dhaka University, Dhaka, Bangladesh. She is a PhD fellow at Bangladesh Medical University, Dhaka, Bangladesh. Hasina Akter has (co)authored more than 20 peer-reviewed articles.

List of Figures

Chapter 7

Chapter 9

Chapter 10

Chapter 16

List of Tables

Chapter 16

Chapter 1
Introduction to Psychiatric Nursing

Hasina Akter and S. M. Yasir Arafat

Abstract Psychiatric nursing plays a vital role in mental healthcare. Mental health is still a largely overlooked issue in Bangladesh, where there is a growing demand for the workforce, highlighting the need for skilled psychiatric nurses. As a specialized field, psychiatric nursing focuses on caring for individuals facing mental health challenges. This chapter introduces the concept of psychiatric nursing and highlights its importance. It also includes ethical and legal issues, like patient rights and confidentiality, in guiding nursing practice. Central to psychiatric care is the psychiatric nursing process, which includes assessment, diagnosis, planning, implementation, and evaluation.

Keywords Psychiatric nursing · Mental health in Bangladesh · Nursing education · Psychiatric care · Nursing in Bangladesh

1 The Concept of Psychiatric Nursing and Its Importance

Psychiatric nursing, also known as *mental health nursing*, is a specialized area of nursing focused on the care of individuals experiencing mental health disorders, emotional disturbances, or psychiatric conditions. It involves the assessment, diagnosis, planning, implementation, and evaluation of care for patients with mental illnesses, in collaboration with the multidisciplinary mental health team. Psychiatric nursing integrates both physical and psychological aspects of care, emphasizing therapeutic communication, crisis intervention, and patient-centered support to promote mental well-being.

H. Akter
Department of Graduate Nursing, Bangladesh Medical University, Dhaka, Bangladesh

S. M. Y. Arafat (✉)
Department of Psychiatry, Bangladesh Specialized Hospital, Dhaka, Bangladesh
e-mail: arafatdmc62@gmail.com

S. M. Y. Arafat and H. Akter (eds.), *Psychiatric Nursing in Bangladesh*, Mental Health Systems and Policy in Low- and Middle-Income Countries,
https://doi.org/10.1007/978-981-95-8501-4_1

Aims

- To provide *safe, empathetic, and evidence-based care* to individuals with mental health conditions.
- To *promote recovery and rehabilitation*, enabling patients to function effectively in society.
- To assist individuals and families in *understanding mental health problems* and adopting positive coping mechanisms.
- To *prevent relapse* and reduce stigma through education and support.

Elements

Psychiatric nursing is rooted in a blend of scientific knowledge and compassionate care (Fig. 1). The essential elements of this specialized field support the comprehensive care of individuals with mental health needs. These elements ensure that care is individualized, ethical, evidence-based, and culturally sensitive, especially in the context of Bangladesh. Establishing a therapeutic relationship is the cornerstone of psychiatric nursing. This involves developing trust, empathy, active listening, and nonjudgmental communication with the patient. Psychiatric nursing plays a role in conducting comprehensive assessments, including mental status examinations (MSE). These assessments assist in diagnosis and planning care according to their unique needs, strengths, and goals. Psychiatric nurses are responsible for formulating, implementing, and evaluating personalized care plans. Administering and managing psychotropic medications is a key component of psychiatric nursing. Nurses educate patients and families on medication use, monitor side effects, and assess therapeutic outcomes. Crisis intervention involves providing immediate and effective support during mental health emergencies, such as suicide risk, acute psychosis, or aggressive behavior. Patient and family education is crucial to recovery. Nurses provide information on the nature of mental illness, treatment adherence, lifestyle modification, and symptom management to the patients as well as the family members. Psychiatric nursing requires close collaboration with other professionals, including psychiatrists, psychologists, social workers, occupational therapists, and the patient's family to work in a team. For example, a nurse in a mental health center joins care planning with a multidisciplinary team. Ethical practice is fundamental to psychiatric nursing. Nurses must uphold patient rights, ensure confidentiality, promote autonomy, and adhere to relevant legal frameworks such as the Mental Health Act, 2018 in Bangladesh. For example, a nurse ensures informed consent and reports misuse of restraints.

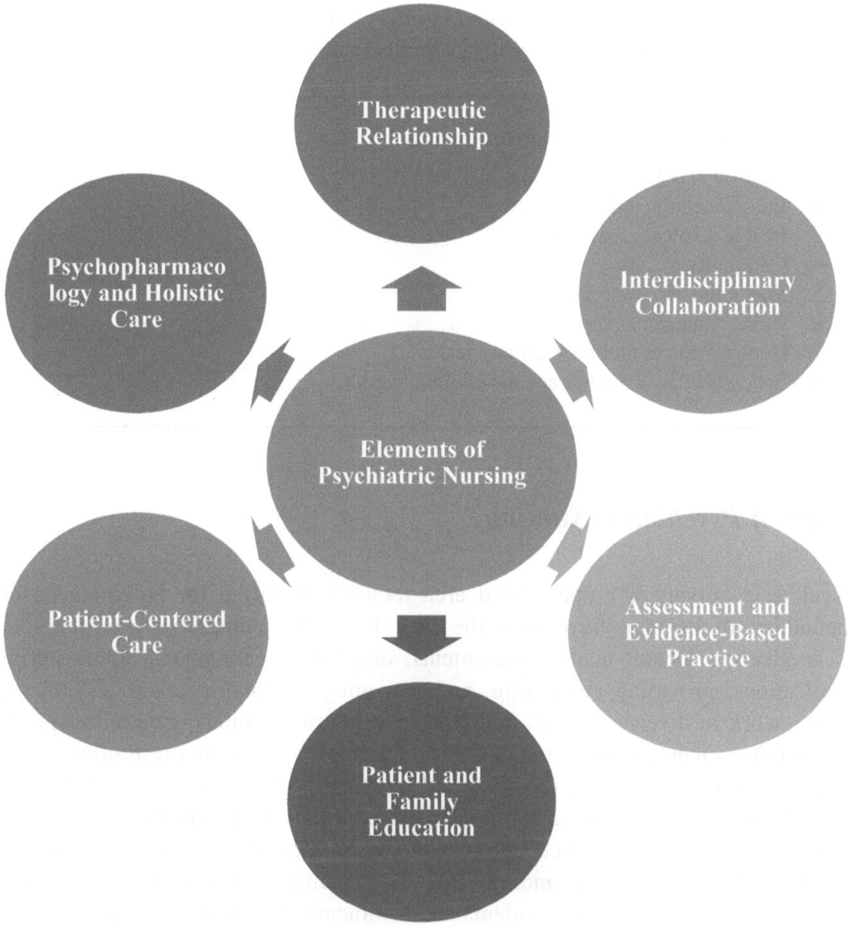

Fig. 1 Elements of psychiatric nursing

Importance of Psychiatric Nursing

Psychiatric nursing focuses on meeting the mental health needs of individuals, families, and communities through holistic as well as person-centered care patterns (Box 1). It addresses physical, emotional, psychological, and social aspects of mental illness, promoting well-being and supporting recovery. Skilled in therapeutic communication and empathy, psychiatric nurses build trust to foster healing. It helps in early detection and timely intervention, preventing complications. Acting as patient advocates, it ensures respectful and dignified care while combating stigma. It ensures care during emergency situations like suicide attempts as well as enduring care for compliance assurance in chronic disorders like schizophrenia. It provides enduring support through counseling, medication adherence, and community reintegration.

Psychiatric nurses educate patients and families to improve mental health awareness and work closely with multidisciplinary teams to develop effective treatment plans.

Box 1: Importance of Psychiatric Nursing

1. Holistic care for mental health patients
2. Early detection and intervention
3. Patient advocacy and support
4. Continuity of care
5. Education and awareness
6. Crisis management
7. Contribution to multidisciplinary teams
8. Specialized skills in therapeutic communication

Scope of Psychiatric Nursing

Psychiatric nursing is a specialized area focused on caring for individuals with mental health disorders throughout the lives. It involves comprehensive roles such as conducting mental health assessments, developing care plans, administering medications, providing counseling, and managing psychiatric crises. Psychiatric nurses work in diverse settings including psychiatric hospitals, general hospitals, community centers, schools, rehabilitation facilities, correctional institutions, non-governmental organizations (NGOs), and tele-health platforms. They extend care beyond hospitals by providing community-based follow-up, promoting mental wellness, preventing relapse, and educating patients, families, and communities to reduce stigma and improve understanding (Box 2). Psychiatric nurses also play important roles in teaching nursing students and healthcare professionals, leading mental health programs, and participating in research to improve care quality. Collaboration with psychiatrists, psychologists, social workers, and other healthcare providers is essential to delivering holistic care. As mental health needs increase globally and in countries like Bangladesh, psychiatric nursing continues to expand, emphasizing advocacy, education, leadership, and evidence-based practice to meet the complex challenges of mental health care.

Box 2: Scope of Psychiatric Nursing

1. Clinical practice
2. Community mental health nursing
3. Mental health promotion and illness prevention
4. Education and teaching role
5. Administrative and leadership role
6. Research and evidence-based practice

7. Collaboration within multidisciplinary teams
8. Settings for psychiatric nursing practice

Principles in Psychiatric Nursing

Psychiatric nursing is founded on essential principles that ensure safe, ethical, and effective care for individuals with mental health conditions. Central to these principles is the acceptance of each patient as a unique individual, treated with dignity and without judgment. Nurses use their communication skills, empathy, and patience as vital therapeutic skills, especially in settings with limited resources. Maintaining professional and goal-directed nurse-patient relationships fosters trust while respecting emotional boundaries. Ensuring a structured and safe environment helps reduce patient anxiety and promotes stability. Continuous observation and accurate reporting of patient behavior support effective treatment planning (Box 3). Nurses gently reorient patients experiencing mental health symptoms (hallucinations and/or delusions) without confrontation, respecting cultural sensitivities. Confidentiality is strictly maintained to build trust and uphold ethical standards. Encouraging patients to take responsibility for daily tasks promotes independence and self-esteem, aiding recovery. Collaboration with multidisciplinary teams enhances holistic care, while nurses' self-awareness and management of their own mental health ensure they provide stable and compassionate care.

Box 3: Principles in Psychiatric Nursing

1. Acceptance of the patient as a unique individual
2. Use of self as a therapeutic tool
3. Maintaining therapeutic nurse-patient relationships
4. Ensuring safety and providing a structured environment
5. Observation and accurate reporting
6. Emphasis on reality orientation
7. Maintaining confidentiality
8. Encouragement of responsibility and independence
9. Multidisciplinary collaboration
10. Awareness of one's own mental health

Roles and Responsibilities of a Psychiatric Nurse

Psychiatric nurses play diverse and vital roles in delivering mental health care. As care provider, they offer holistic care addressing physical, emotional, and psychological needs by administering medications, monitoring side effects, and assisting with daily activities (Box 4). They act as communicators by building therapeutic relationships through active listening and empathy, offering support to patients who feel isolated or fearful. As educators, psychiatric nurses help patients and families understand mental illnesses, medications, and coping strategies, such as conducting family sessions to reduce stigma about depression. In their advocacy role, they uphold patients' rights and dignity, often protecting confidentiality even in challenging cultural contexts. Nurses are also observers and reporters, monitoring patient behavior and documenting symptoms to inform treatment decisions—for example, reporting suicidal thoughts to the psychiatrist.

During psychiatric emergencies, they serve as crisis managers by using de-escalation techniques to ensure safety. As rehabilitation facilitators, they support patients in regaining independence and reintegrating into society, encouraging activities like vocational training post-discharge (Box 5). In multidisciplinary teams, they collaborate with psychiatrists, psychologists, and social workers during ward rounds to ensure coordinated care. Although not professional therapists, they offer emotional support as counselors under supervision, helping patients process grief or trauma. Their emerging role as researchers contributes to improving care practices. Psychiatric nurses also act as cultural mediators by respecting patients' beliefs and practices, including observing prayer times or fasting during Ramadan. Lastly, as mental health promoters, they raise awareness and reduce stigma through community outreach, such as organizing stress management sessions in schools or rural areas. These varied roles reflect the critical importance of psychiatric nurses in advancing mental health care and supporting recovery across diverse settings.

Box 4: Roles and Responsibilities of a Psychiatric Nurse

1. Care provider
2. Communicator
3. Educator
4. Advocate
5. Observer and reporter
6. Crisis manager
7. Rehabilitation facilitator
8. Team member
9. Counselor
10. Researcher
11. Cultural mediator
12. Mental health promoter

Box 5: Quality of Psychiatric Nurses

Empathy and compassion

- Understands the emotions and problems of the patient
- Provides care with kindness, patience, and non-judgmental support
- Builds strong therapeutic relationships with the patients

Strong communication skills

- Listens actively and responds appropriately
- Uses therapeutic communication techniques to foster trust
- Effectively conveys complex medical and psychological information

Emotional resilience and patience

- Handles stressful and emotionally challenging situations calmly
- Maintains professionalism under pressure and during crises
- Avoids burnout through self-care and emotional regulation

Critical thinking and problem-solving

- Assesses complex mental health conditions effectively
- Analyzes patient behaviors to make informed clinical decisions
- Quickly adapts interventions to changing patient needs

Ethical and professional conduct

- Maintains strict patient confidentiality and privacy
- Adheres to ethical nursing guidelines and legal frameworks
- Respects patient autonomy and informed consent

Teamwork and interdisciplinary collaboration

- Works effectively with psychiatrists, psychologists, social workers, and caregivers
- Coordinates care plans with interdisciplinary healthcare teams
- Contributes to a supportive and inclusive care environment

Continuous learning and adaptability

- Stays updated on advancements in psychiatric care and treatments
- Adapts to new therapies, medications, and patient care approaches
- Participates in ongoing training, research, and professional development

Strong observation and assessment skills

- Identifies early signs of deterioration in mental health conditions
- Monitors medication effects, side effects, and therapeutic responses
- Documents and reports changes in patient behavior accurately

Advocacy for patients' rights and well-being

- Protects and supports the rights of patients with mental health conditions
- Ensures that patients receive appropriate and humane care
- Addresses stigma and promotes mental health awareness

Ability to manage crisis and de-escalation

- Uses crisis intervention techniques to prevent harm
- Implements de-escalation strategies during aggressive or violent situations
- Ensures a safe and therapeutic environment for all patients

Functions of Psychiatric Nurses in Various Settings

Psychiatric nurses serve essential functions across various healthcare settings, each tailored to the needs of the environment and population they serve. In inpatient psychiatric hospitals, they manage acute mental health conditions by administering medications, implementing behavior modification programs, providing therapeutic support, and closely monitoring patients' mental status. In outpatient psychiatric units, nurses assist psychiatrists during consultations, educate patients about medication adherence, follow up with discharged individuals, and provide psychoeducation and counseling support. Community mental health centers rely on psychiatric nurses to lead awareness campaigns, identify at-risk individuals, deliver basic mental health services, and conduct home visits. In the general hospitals with psychiatric wards, psychiatric nurses care for patients with both physical and mental health issues, provide crisis intervention, educate general staff on mental health, and collaborate with physicians for integrated care. In schools and educational institutions, they identify behavioral concerns, offer mental health first aid, make necessary referrals, and promote mental well-being through health education. In prisons and rehabilitation centers, psychiatric nurses perform mental health assessments for inmates or recovering addicts, monitor treatment compliance, support psychological rehabilitation, and coordinate with legal and social services. In NGOs and outreach programs, psychiatric nurses contribute to mobile mental health clinics, offer culturally sensitive counseling, educate underserved communities, and provide care in disaster-affected regions. Lastly, in psychiatric research and education, nurses engage in research projects, train junior staff, promote evidence-based practices, and assist in creating training materials. These diverse roles highlight the adaptability and importance of psychiatric nurses in improving mental health outcomes across all sectors of society.

Rights of a Psychiatric Patient and Psychiatric Nurse

Rights of a Psychiatric Patient

Psychiatric patients, like all individuals, are entitled to fundamental human rights that uphold their dignity, autonomy, and well-being (Box 6). Every psychiatric patient has the right to be treated with dignity and respect, regardless of their diagnosis. They are entitled to provide informed consent, meaning they must be given clear information about treatment options and allowed to make voluntary decisions. Confidentiality must be maintained, with personal health information only disclosed when legally or ethically justified. Patients also have the right to receive appropriate and evidence-based mental health care, as well as the right to refuse treatment unless they are legally declared incompetent or pose a threat to themselves or others. Ensuring safety is another essential right, with patients needing protection from abuse, neglect, or exploitation. Psychiatric patients should be actively involved in care planning decisions, promoting autonomy and collaboration. They also have the right to communicate with family members, legal representatives, and spiritual advisors, which supports emotional and legal well-being. Access to legal representation is especially important during cases of involuntary admission or treatment. Importantly, patients should have the right to live in the least restrictive environment, ideally within the community, rather than being institutionalized without necessity.

Box 6: Key Rights of Psychiatric Patients

Dignity and respect
Informed consent
Confidentiality
Receive treatment
Refuse treatment
Safety and protection
Participate in care planning
Communication
Legal representation
Live in the community

Rights of a Psychiatric Nurse

One of the primary rights is the right to a safe working environment, where risks of violence or harm from patients are minimized through proper security measures and support systems. Nurses also deserve professional respect, recognizing their expertise and contributions as essential members of the healthcare team. Access to adequate resources, proper training, and supervision is vital to enable nurses to deliver quality care, while fair and timely compensation acknowledges their hard work and commitment (Box 7). Legal protection is crucial for nurses performing their duties within professional boundaries, shielding them from undue legal consequences. Opportunities for continuing education should be provided to keep nurses updated on best practices and emerging trends in mental health care. Additionally, psychiatric nurses must have the right to voice concerns regarding patient care or workplace issues without fear of retaliation, fostering transparency and safety. The right to self-care is equally important, allowing nurses to manage their own mental and physical health, which is vital in such a demanding field. Lastly, professional autonomy must be respected, enabling nurses to make informed judgments within their scope of practice, particularly in clinical decision-making. Upholding these rights not only protects nurses but also strengthens the mental healthcare system by promoting ethical practice, reducing burnout, and ensuring high standards of care.

Box 7: Key Rights of Psychiatric Nurses Right to-

Safe working environment
Professional respect
Adequate resources and support
Fair compensation
Legal protection
Continuing education
Voice concerns
Self-care
Professional autonomy

Psychiatric Nursing Skills

One of the core competencies is therapeutic communication, which involves building trust and rapport with patients through empathy, active listening, and nonjudgmental attitude. Equally important are observation and assessment skills, which help nurses detect changes in behavior, mood, and cognitive functioning, guiding timely interventions. Psychosocial intervention skills enable nurses to facilitate group therapy, offer individual support, and teach coping strategies that promote recovery (Box 8). Administering psychotropic medications safely and educating patients about their treatment is another vital role, requiring strong pharmacological knowledge. In psychiatric emergencies, crisis intervention and de-escalation techniques are essential to manage aggression, suicidal behavior, or acute psychosis while maintaining a safe environment. Cultural sensitivity is also crucial, as nurses must respect the diverse beliefs and practices of patients. Effective documentation ensures accurate records of patient progress and nursing interventions, supporting legal and clinical standards. Psychiatric nurses must also collaborate with interdisciplinary teams such as psychiatrists, psychologists, and social workers to provide holistic care. Additionally, educating patients and families about mental illness and available resources helps reduce stigma and empowers recovery. Finally, self-awareness and emotional resilience are necessary for maintaining professional boundaries, managing stress, and sustaining the nurse's well-being.

Box 8: Key Psychiatric Nursing Skills

Therapeutic communication skills

- Build trust and rapport using active listening and empathy
- Use non-judgmental language to encourage expression

Observation and assessment skills

- Monitor behavior, mood, and thought patterns
- Identify early signs of improvement or deterioration

Psychosocial intervention skills

- Support individual, group, and family therapy
- Provide psychoeducation and teach basic coping strategies

Medication administration skills

- Administer psychotropic drugs
- Monitor side effects and educate on adherence

Crisis intervention skills

- Handle emergencies like aggression or suicide risk
- Use de-escalation and ensure safety

Cultural sensitivity and competence

- Respect cultural beliefs in care delivery
- Address mental health stigma in communities

Documentation skills

- Keep proper and confidential records
- Document assessments, care, and outcomes

Teamwork and interdisciplinary collaboration

- Coordinate with other team members
- Contribute to team-based care planning

Patient and family education skills

- Educate on illness, treatment, and medications
- Guide on available community support

Self-awareness and emotional resilience

- Manage stress and maintain boundaries
- Practice self-care to stay emotionally healthy

2 Concept of Mental Health

The World Health Organization (WHO) defines, mental health is a state of well-being in which an individual realizes their own abilities, can cope with the normal stresses of life, can work productively, and is able to contribute to their community. It involves emotional, psychological, and social well-being, affecting how people think, feel, and act. Good mental health allows individuals to maintain fulfilling relationships, adapt to change, and deal with adversity. It is not merely the absence of mental illness but includes the presence of positive characteristics such as resilience, self-esteem, and emotional regulation. Mental health is shaped by a range of factors including genetics, life experiences, family environment, and social and cultural influences. Maintaining mental health requires a balance in various aspects of life, including physical health, relationships, work, and recreation (Fig. 2).

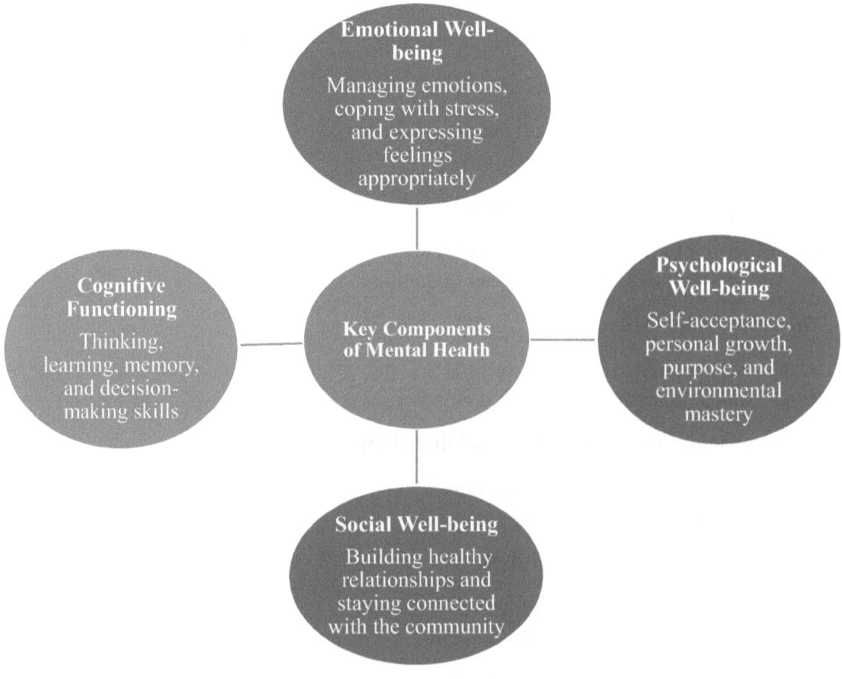

Fig. 2 Key components of mental health

Key Components of Mental Health

Importance of Mental Health

Good mental health is essential for overall well-being as it influences physical health, emotional stability, and the ability to manage daily stress. It plays a vital role in enhancing the quality of life by supporting effective functioning in relationships, work, and recreational activities. Mental well-being is also closely tied to productivity and performance, contributing to creativity and efficiency in academic and professional settings (Box 9). Moreover, mental and physical health are interconnected—poor mental health can lead to or worsen chronic physical illnesses. On a broader level, mentally healthy individuals positively impact their communities by fostering social harmony and economic stability. Early attention to mental health concerns allows for timely intervention, preventing more severe disorders and easing pressure on healthcare systems. Additionally, good mental health helps build resilience, enabling people to cope effectively with life's challenges and bounce back from adversity.

Box 9: Importance of Mental Health

- Overall well-being
- Quality of life
- Productivity and performance
- Physical health connection
- Community and social impact
- Prevention and early intervention
- Resilience and coping

Mental Illness

Mental illness refers to a wide range of mental health conditions that affect a person's thinking, feeling, mood, behavior, and ability to relate to others and function in daily life. These conditions can be mild or severe, temporary or long-lasting, and may include disorders such as depression, anxiety, schizophrenia, bipolar disorder, and obsessive-compulsive disorder. Mental illness is caused by a complex interplay of genetic, biological, psychological, and environmental factors. It can disrupt personal relationships, work performance, and overall quality of life.

Mental Disorder

The *Diagnostic and Statistical Manual of Mental Disorders* (DSM-5) mentioned that "a mental disorder is a syndrome characterized by clinically significant disturbance in an individual's cognition, emotion regulation, or behavior that reflects a dysfunction in the psychological, biological, or developmental processes underlying mental functioning."

Common Mental Health Disorders

The *International Classification of Diseases*, 11th Revision (ICD-11), developed by WHO, provides a comprehensive classification system for all diseases, including mental health disorders (Box 10). It organizes mental, behavioral, and neurodevelopmental disorders into specific categories based on symptoms, clinical presentation, and etiology.

Box 10: Common Mental Health Disorders as Per ICD-11 Classification

- **Schizophrenia and psychotic disorders**—Schizophrenia, schizoaffective disorder, delusional disorder, catatonia.
- **Mood disorders**—Bipolar disorder, major depressive disorder, dysthymia, cyclothymia.
- **Anxiety disorders**—Generalized Anxiety Disorder (GAD), panic disorder, phobias, agoraphobia, separation anxiety.
- **Obsessive-compulsive disorders**—OCD, hoarding disorder, body dysmorphic disorder.
- **Stress-related disorders**—Post-traumatic stress disorder (PTSD), acute stress reaction, adjustment disorder.
- **Dissociative disorders**—Dissociative amnesia, identity disorder, depersonalization.
- **Somatic symptom disorders**—Somatic symptom disorder, conversion disorder, illness anxiety.
- **Eating disorders**—Anorexia, bulimia, binge-eating disorder, pica.
- **Substance use disorders**—Alcohol, opioids, stimulants, gambling, gaming disorder.
- **Neurodevelopmental disorders**—Autism, Attention deficit hyperactivity disorder (ADHD), intellectual disability, learning disorders.
- **Neurocognitive disorders**—Delirium, dementia (Alzheimer's, Parkinson's).
- **Child and adolescent disorders**—Conduct disorder, Oppositional Defiant Disorder (ODD), attachment disorders.
- **Sexual and gender disorders**—Sexual dysfunctions, paraphilia, gender incongruence.

Characteristics of Mentally Healthy and Mentally Ill Individuals

Mentally healthy individuals generally display emotional stability, effectively managing their emotions, coping with stress, and showing resilience in difficult situations. They possess a balanced self-image, demonstrating self-acceptance and confidence, which contributes to their ability to build and maintain positive, healthy relationships. Their decision-making is rational and well-informed, and they typically use constructive coping strategies to handle challenges. Adaptable by nature, mentally healthy people are open to change and approach life with a realistic and optimistic perspective. They remain socially engaged, participate in activities, and manage daily responsibilities such as work, school, and self-care effectively. Importantly, they have awareness of their emotional state and are willing to seek help when needed.

In contrast, individuals with mental illness often struggle with emotional instability, experiencing intense mood swings, anxiety, or emotional distress (Table 1). They may suffer from low self-esteem, self-criticism, and feelings of worthlessness, which can negatively affect their relationships, leading to isolation, irritability, or conflict. Their ability to make decisions may be impaired due to poor concentration, memory issues, or distorted thinking. They may rely on harmful coping mechanisms such as substance abuse or self-harm. Mentally ill individuals can find it difficult to adapt to changes, often exhibiting rigid thinking or paranoia. Their outlook on life may be pessimistic or unrealistic, and they tend to withdraw from social interactions, which can lead to further isolation. Daily functioning, including work and self-care, becomes challenging, and they may lack awareness of their mental condition or deny the need for help. In more severe cases, they may experience suicidal thoughts or engage in self-harming behavior.

Table 1 Characteristics of mentally healthy and mentally ill individuals

Mentally healthy individuals	Mentally ill individuals
Emotional stability	Emotional instability
Positive self-image	Negative self-image
Healthy relationships	Relationship difficulties
Rational decision-making	Impaired decision-making
Constructive coping skills	Maladaptive coping mechanisms
Adaptability	Poor adaptability
Optimistic outlook	Pessimistic perspective
Social engagement	Social withdrawal
Effective daily functioning	Daily functioning challenges
Mental health awareness	Lack of insight
Low risk of suicidal thoughts	Risk of suicidal behavior

3 Determinants of Mental Health and Mental Illness

Mental health and mental illness are shaped by a complex interplay of biological, psychological, social, environmental, lifestyle, and political-economic factors. Biological factors such as genetics, brain chemistry, and hormonal changes play a significant role; for instance, a family history of mental illness or chemical imbalances in neurotransmitters can increase vulnerability. Chronic physical illnesses and life stages like puberty or menopause can also influence mental health (Fig. 3). Psychological factors include individual personality traits, coping mechanisms, and experiences of trauma. People with low self-esteem, poor stress management skills, or a history of abuse or loss are more susceptible to mental health challenges. Social factors such as supportive relationships, socioeconomic status, and cultural beliefs significantly impact mental well-being. Individuals with strong social connections are more resilient, while poverty, unemployment, and stigma can contribute to mental illness. Environmental factors also matter; safe housing, manageable work demands, and a secure community promote mental stability, whereas poor living conditions and exposure to violence increase psychological stress. Lifestyle choices—including diet, exercise, sleep, and substance use directly affect mental health. A nutritious diet, regular physical activity, and adequate sleep can improve emotional resilience, while substance abuse and poor lifestyle habits worsen mental health outcomes. Lastly, political and economic factors such as healthcare access, job security, and economic policies influence the availability of mental health services and overall well-being. Understanding these determinants is essential for promoting mental health, preventing illness, and designing effective interventions.

4 Mental Health Illness Continuum

The mental health illness continuum is a framework that illustrates the spectrum of mental health, ranging from optimal mental well-being to severe mental illness. This model emphasizes that mental health exists on a continuum rather than being strictly categorized into "healthy" or "ill" states (Fig. 4). Understanding this continuum helps to recognize the varying degrees of mental health and the potential for change and recovery.

5 Cultural and Socioeconomic Factors Related to Mental Health Care

Cultural and socioeconomic factors play a significant role in shaping mental health care access, attitudes, and outcomes (Fig. 5). Cultural factors such as stigma and traditional beliefs often lead to the underreporting of mental illness and delays in seeking

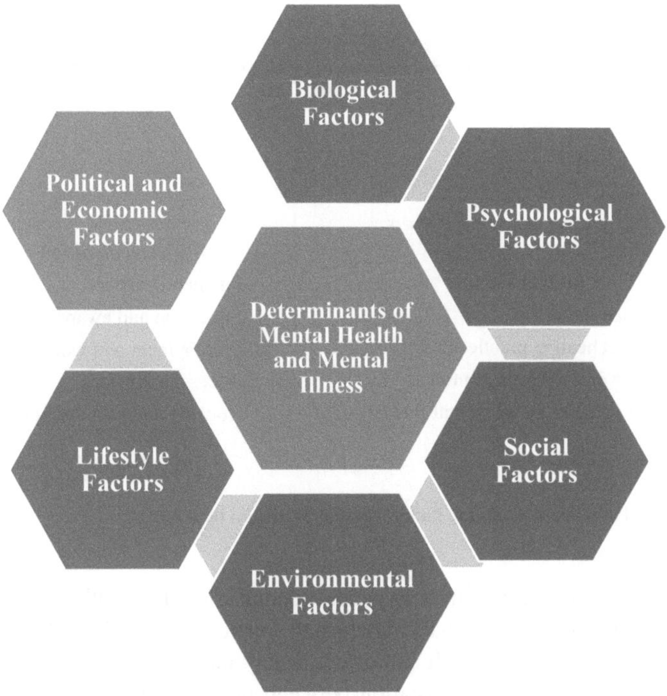

Fig. 3 Determinants of mental health and mental illness

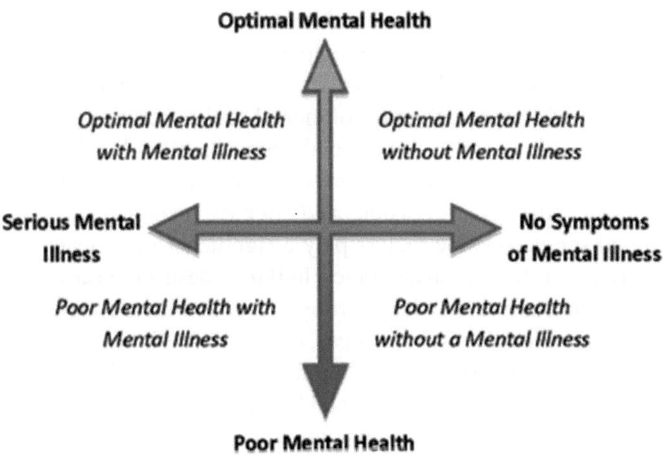

Fig. 4 Mental health illness continuum

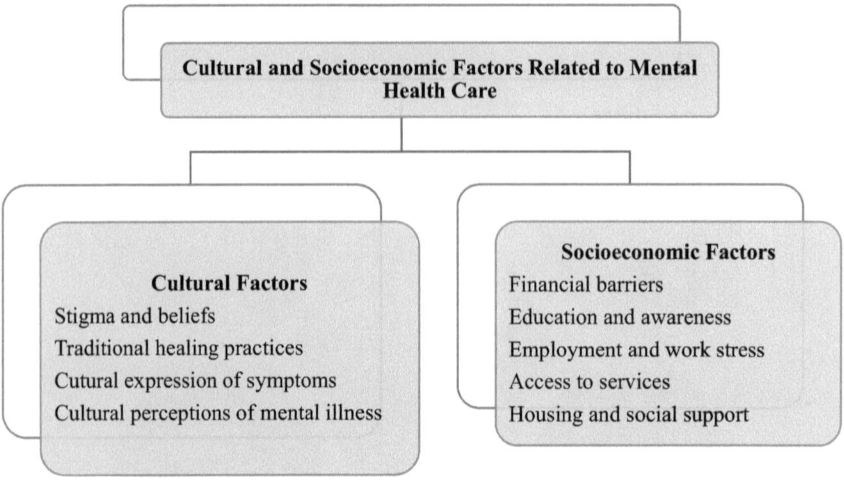

Fig. 5 Cultural and socioeconomic factors related to mental health care

treatment, as some communities associate mental disorders with shame or moral failure. In many cases, individuals may turn to spiritual or traditional healers instead of medical professionals, which can affect timely and appropriate care. Language barriers further hinder communication between patients and providers, impacting diagnosis, treatment adherence, and recovery. On the other hand, socioeconomic factors like financial limitations restrict access to mental health services. Low levels of education and awareness about mental health contribute to widespread misconceptions and reluctance to seek help. Employment-related stress and job insecurity also increase the risk of mental health issues. Furthermore, people living in rural or low-income areas often face a shortage of mental health facilities and professionals. Poor housing conditions and lack of social support further heighten vulnerability to mental health disorders. Addressing these cultural and socioeconomic barriers is essential to ensure equitable, accessible, and effective mental health care.

Cultural and socioeconomic factors play a significant role in shaping access to mental health care, attitudes, and outcomes. In Bangladesh, cultural stigma and traditional beliefs often lead to the underreporting of mental illness and delays in seeking treatment. For example, in many rural areas, mental illness is still viewed as a sign of spiritual possession or punishment, leading families to seek help from traditional or spiritual healers rather than qualified mental health professionals. This delays timely diagnosis and treatment. Language and communication barriers are also common in Bangladesh, especially where local languages dominate, and mental health literacy is low. In remote areas, patients may not understand medical terminology or may feel intimidated by formal healthcare settings. This affects communication, trust, and adherence to treatment. On the other hand, socioeconomic challenges further limit access to mental health services. In urban slums like those in Korail (Dhaka) or Halishahar (Chattogram), many families live below the poverty line and cannot afford private psychiatric care. Public mental health facilities are scarce, and health insurance coverage for mental illnesses is almost nonexistent. In rural Upazilas, there are often no psychiatrists or clinical psychologists available, leaving general practitioners or untrained personnel to manage mental health cases. Additionally, low levels of education and awareness lead to widespread myths, such as the belief that depression is "just a weakness" or that psychiatric medications cause madness. Job insecurity, especially among garment workers and unemployed youth, contributes to high levels of anxiety, depression, and even suicide. Overcrowded housing, lack of clean-living environments, and minimal social support systems—common in both urban and rural poor communities—further increase vulnerability to mental health issues. Addressing these barriers through community-based mental health services, awareness campaigns, school programs, and increased government investment is essential to ensure equitable, accessible, and effective mental health care in Bangladesh.

6 Ethical and Legal Issues in Psychiatric Nursing

Ethical and legal issues are central to psychiatric nursing, as nurses often work with vulnerable individuals who may be unable to fully advocate for themselves. Ethical principles such as autonomy, confidentiality, informed consent, beneficence, and non-maleficence must guide every aspect of care (Boxes 11 and 12). Psychiatric nurses are responsible for respecting patients' rights, ensuring their dignity, and promoting voluntary treatment whenever possible. However, situations such as involuntary admissions, use of restraints, or treating patients who lack decision-making capacity often present ethical dilemmas. Legally, nurses must adhere to mental health laws and regulations, such as the Mental Health Act, 2018, in Bangladesh, which outlines the rights of individuals with mental illness and provides guidelines for their care. Breaching confidentiality, failing to obtain proper consent, or using unethical practices can lead to serious legal consequences. Therefore, psychiatric nurses must stay informed about current laws, hospital policies, and ethical standards to ensure safe, respectful, and lawful care for all patients.

Box 11: Ethical Issues

1. **Autonomy**: Respecting the patient's right to make informed decisions about their own care.
2. **Confidentiality**: Protecting the privacy of patient information all times.
3. **Informed consent**: Ensuring patients understand and agree to treatment voluntarily.
4. **Beneficence**: Acting in the best interest of the patient to promote well-being.
5. **Non-maleficence**: Avoiding harm to the patient during care and treatment.

Box 12: Legal Issues

- **Mental health laws**: Following legal frameworks such as the Mental Health Act, 2018, in Bangladesh.
- **Patient rights**: Upholding rights related to dignity, freedom, and fair treatment.
- **Use of restraints**: Applying physical or chemical restraints only under legal and ethical guidelines.
- **Involuntary admission**: Admitting patients against their will only when legally justified.
- **Legal accountability**: Nurses can be held legally responsible for violating laws or patient rights.
- **Documentation**: Accurate and legal record-keeping is essential for accountability and patient safety.

7 Psychiatric Nursing Process

The psychiatric nursing process is a structured and evidence-based method used to deliver comprehensive and individualized care to patients with mental health conditions. It follows five key steps: *assessment, diagnosis, planning, implementation, and evaluation.* In the *assessment* phase, psychiatric nurses gather detailed information about the patient's mental, emotional, physical, and social health through interviews, observations, and reports. This helps in identifying symptoms, coping strategies, and risk factors such as suicidal thoughts or substance use. The next step is *diagnosis*, where nurses analyze the symptoms and use standardized criteria like the DSM-5 to identify psychiatric disorders and formulate nursing diagnoses, such as ineffective coping or risk for self-harm. In the *planning* phase, a patient-centered care plan is developed in collaboration with the patient, family, and healthcare team. This includes setting measurable goals, prioritizing needs, and selecting evidence-based interventions. The *implementation* phase involves putting the care plan into action by administering medications, providing therapy, offering psychoeducation, and engaging in therapeutic communication while monitoring the patient's responses. Finally, the *evaluation* phase assesses the effectiveness of interventions. Nurses review the patient's progress toward the goals, reassess symptoms and behaviors, and modify the care plan as needed.

The psychiatric nursing process involves five key steps

1. **Assessment**

   - **Objective:** Collect comprehensive data about the patient's mental, physical, emotional, and social health.
   - **Actions:**

     – Gather information through interviews, observations, physical assessments, and reports from family members or other healthcare providers.

- Assess symptoms of mental illness (e.g., mood, behavior, cognitive function) and the patient's coping mechanisms, strengths, and needs.
- Identify risk factors such as suicidal ideation, substance use, or history of trauma.

2. **Diagnosis**

- **Objective:** Identify the mental health issues and conditions that need to be addressed.
- **Actions:**

  – Analyze the assessment data to identify problems or needs.

- Use diagnostic criteria (e.g., DSM-5) to categorize mental health conditions and label psychiatric disorders.
- Formulate nursing diagnoses that reflect the patient's primary issues (e.g., risk for self-harm, ineffective coping, impaired social interaction).

3. **Planning**

- **Objective:** Develop a patient-specific care plan with measurable goals and interventions.
- **Actions:**

  – Collaborate with the patient, their family, and the healthcare team to establish short-term and long-term goals.
  – Prioritize the patient's needs based on severity and urgency.
  – Choose evidence-based interventions (e.g., medications, therapy) that will help meet the established goals.
  – Identify resources and support systems that can assist the patient in their recovery.

4. **Implementation**

- **Objective:** Carry out the planned interventions to address the identified problems.
- **Actions:**

  – Provide direct care, including administering medications, providing therapy (individual/group), and offering psychoeducation.
  – Monitor the patient's response to interventions, ensuring they are safe and appropriate.
  – Adjust interventions based on the patient's evolving needs.
  – Engage in therapeutic communication, helping the patient express feelings and concerns while providing emotional support.

5. **Evaluation**

- **Objective:** Assess the effectiveness of the interventions and adjust the care plan as needed.

- **Actions:**
  - Evaluate the patient's progress toward achieving the set goals.
  - Assess changes in symptoms, behavior, and overall functioning.
  - Collaborate with the healthcare team to determine if the goals were met, partially met, or unmet.
- Modify the care plan, incorporating new interventions or altering existing ones based on the evaluation.

MSE

The **MSE** is a structured assessment used by healthcare professionals to evaluate a patient's current mental functioning. It covers different aspects of mental health, including appearance, behavior, mood, speech, thought, perception, cognition, and insight.

1. **Appearance and Behavior**
   - General appearance: Observations of grooming, hygiene, clothing, and physical condition.
   - Facial appearance: Expression, eye contact, and emotional responsiveness.
   - Rapport: The ease of interaction between the patient and the examiner.
   - Posture and movement: Body posture, gestures, and any signs of agitation or retardation.
   - Social behavior: Ability to engage appropriately in social situations.
   - Motor behavior: Observations of psychomotor activity, restlessness, or slow movements.
   - Oddity of behavior: Presence of bizarre or unusual behaviors.
2. **Mood and Affect**
   - Nature: The patient's predominant emotional state (e.g., depressed, anxious, euphoric).
   - Change: Stability or fluctuation in mood.
   - Congruence: Whether the mood matches the situation or thought content.
3. **Speech**
   - Rate and quantity: Speed and amount of speech (e.g., slow, rapid, pressured, reduced).
   - Volume and tone: Loudness, pitch, or monotone speech.
   - Flow and rhythm: Fluency, coherence, and presence of interruptions or stuttering.
   - Oddity of speech: Unusual speech patterns, neologisms, or echolalia.

4. **Thought**
   - Stream: The rate of thought production (e.g., flight of ideas, poverty of thought).
   - Possession: Awareness of one's own thoughts (e.g., thought insertion, withdrawal).
   - Form: Logical or disorganized thought processes (e.g., tangential, circumstantial).
   - Content: Presence of delusions, obsessions, or preoccupations.
5. **Perception**
   - Hallucinations: False sensory experiences (e.g., auditory, visual, tactile).
   - Illusions: Misinterpretation of actual stimuli.
6. **Cognition**
   - Consciousness: Awareness of self and surroundings (e.g., alert, drowsy, stupor).
   - Orientation: Awareness of time, place, and person.
   - Attention and concentration: Ability to focus and sustain mental effort.
   - Memory: Immediate, short-term, and long-term recall.
   - Intelligence: General intellectual abilities, comprehension, and reasoning skills.
7. **Judgment and Insight**
   - Judgment: The ability to make sound decisions in daily life.
   - Insight: Awareness of one's mental health condition and need for treatment

8 Community Mental Health Nursing

Community mental health nursing is a specialized field that emphasizes the promotion of mental well-being, prevention of mental illness, and delivery of care to individuals with mental health disorders within their own communities. It adopts a holistic and proactive approach, focusing not only on treating existing conditions but also on identifying and addressing risk factors early. Community mental health nurses work in diverse settings such as homes, schools, clinics, and community centers, making mental health services more accessible, especially to underserved populations. This practice recognizes that mental health is shaped by a combination of social, economic, cultural, and environmental influences. By integrating mental health care into community-based systems, this approach helps reduce stigma, encourages early intervention, and fosters supportive networks that promote recovery and resilience.

Principles of Community Mental Health Nursing

The principles of community mental health nursing provide a foundation for delivering effective and compassionate care within the community setting (Box 13). *Holistic care* is central, as it addresses not only the psychological needs but also the physical, social, and spiritual well-being of individuals, recognizing that mental health is deeply interconnected with overall health. An emphasis is placed on *prevention and promotion*, aiming to reduce the incidence of mental illness through early intervention, education, and public awareness programs that highlight mental health as a vital part of public health. *Client-centered care* ensures that individuals and their families are actively involved in decision-making and care planning, with interventions tailored to meet their unique needs and preferences. Another key principle is *collaboration and interdisciplinary approach*, where community mental health nurses coordinate with a range of professionals—such as psychologists, psychiatrists, social workers, and local organizations—to provide integrated and comprehensive care. *Cultural competence* is also essential, as it ensures care is respectful of and responsive to cultural beliefs and practices regarding mental health. A*ccessibility and outreach* focus on delivering mental health services to all segments of the population, particularly marginalized and underserved groups, by implementing community-based initiatives and outreach programs.

Box 13: Principles of Community Mental Health Nursing

1. Holistic care
2. Prevention and promotion
3. Client-centered care
4. Collaboration and interdisciplinary approach.
5. Cultural competence
6. Accessibility and outreach

Roles of Community Mental Health Nurses

Community mental health nurses play diverse and vital roles in promoting mental well-being and addressing mental health needs at the community level (Fig. 6). One of their key responsibilities is *assessment and diagnosis*, where they conduct mental health screenings, evaluate individuals' psychological status, and assess the effectiveness of interventions within the community. They are also active in *education and advocacy*, raising awareness about mental health issues, working to reduce stigma, and advocating for individuals' rights and equitable access to services. Through *therapeutic interventions*, these nurses provide evidence-based support such as counseling, crisis intervention, and facilitation of support groups for individuals and families. In their role as *case managers,* they coordinate care for clients with complex

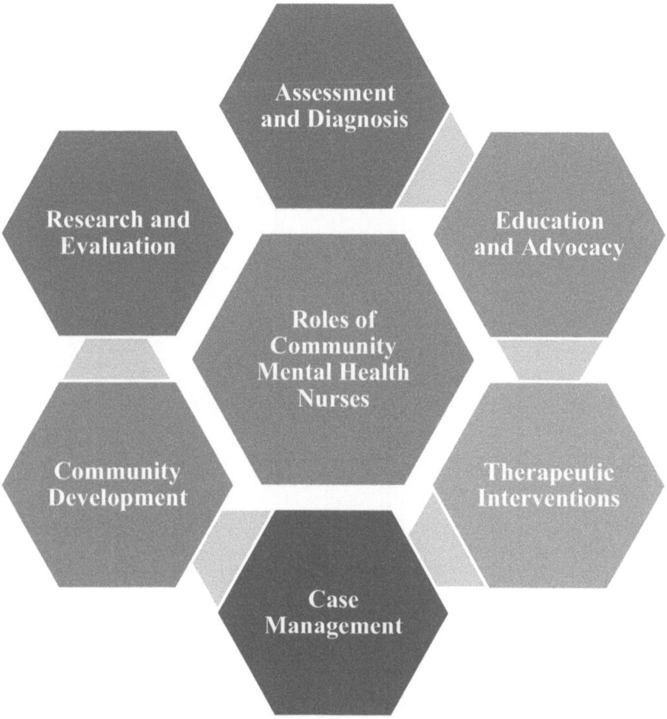

Fig. 6 Roles of community mental health nurses

mental health needs, ensuring that appropriate services, referrals, and follow-up support are in place. Community mental health nurses are also involved in *community development* by building mental health awareness, establishing local support networks, and collaborating with community partners to strengthen mental health resources. Lastly, they contribute to *research and evaluation* by participating in studies that assess the impact and effectiveness of mental health programs, helping to shape policies and refine practices in the field.

Challenges in Community Mental Health Nursing in Bangladesh

Community mental health nursing faces several challenges that can impact the delivery and effectiveness of care (Fig. 7). *Stigma and discrimination* remain significant barriers, as negative perceptions about mental illness often discourage individuals from seeking help or engaging with services. This stigma can also affect how communities support mental health initiatives. *Limited resources* pose another major challenge, with many community mental health programs operating under

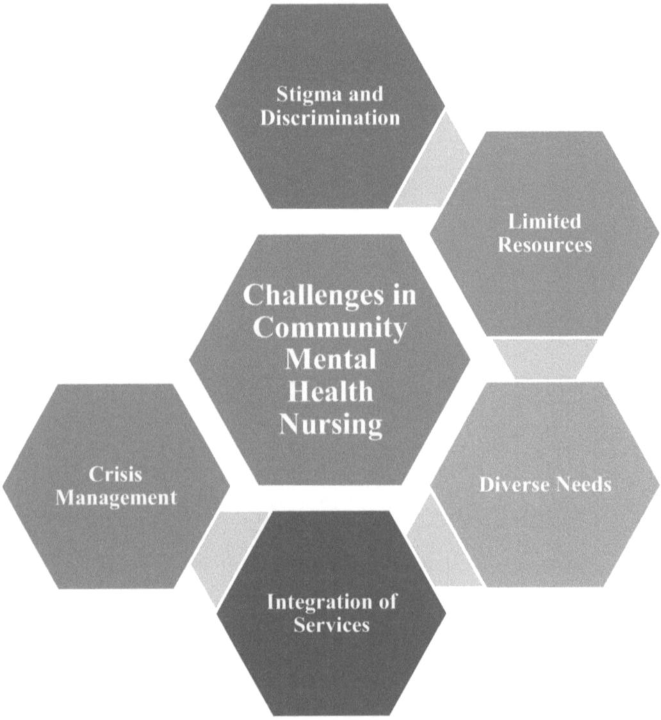

Fig. 7 Challenges in community mental health nursing

constraints such as inadequate funding, staffing shortages, and a lack of accessible treatment facilities. The *diverse needs* of individuals in the community further complicate care, requiring nurses to demonstrate cultural competence and adapt services to accommodate differences in expression, beliefs, and socioeconomic backgrounds. Another difficulty lies in the *integration of services*, as coordinating care across various healthcare providers, social services, and community organizations is often complex—especially for clients with multiple or chronic conditions. Additionally, *crisis management* in community settings can be demanding, as it requires rapid, well-coordinated responses and immediate access to resources, which may not always be available. Addressing these challenges is essential to improving mental health outcomes and ensuring equitable, effective care at the community level.

Interventions in Community Mental Health Nursing

Interventions in community mental health nursing are designed to promote mental wellness, provide support, and ensure accessible care for individuals within their communities (Fig. 8). *Public awareness campaigns* play a crucial role by educating

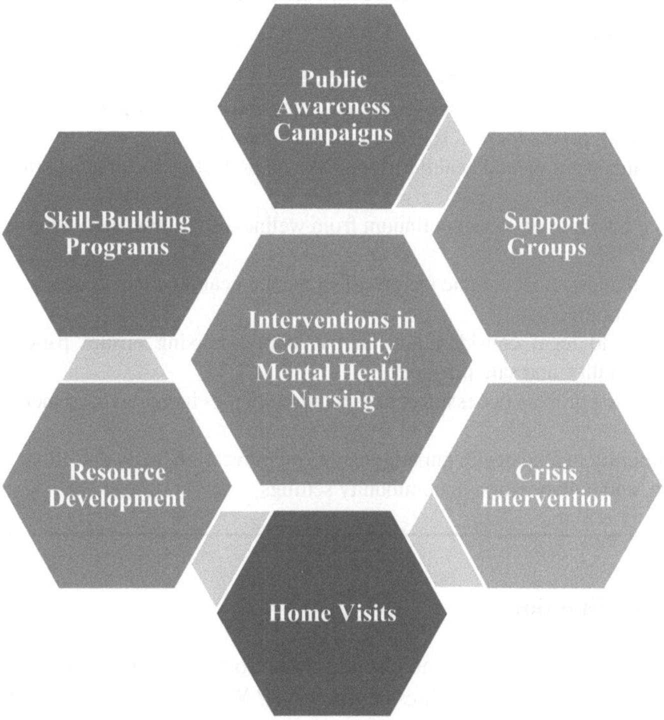

Fig. 8 Interventions in community mental health nursing

the public about mental health, reducing stigma, and informing people about available services and support systems. *Support groups* offer safe spaces for individuals with mental health conditions and their families to share experiences, exchange coping strategies, and foster a sense of community.

In times of acute need, *crisis intervention* ensures that individuals facing mental health emergencies receive immediate support, including connection to emergency services and resources for stabilization. *Home visits* are another vital intervention, especially for those who face barriers like limited mobility or social isolation, allowing nurses to provide care in a comfortable and familiar environment. *Resource development* involves working with community partners to build or expand mental health services, such as helplines, shelters, and accessible outpatient care. Lastly, *skill-building programs* empower individuals with practical tools to manage stress, build resilience, and maintain mental well-being, ultimately strengthening the overall mental health of the community.

Take Home Message

- Psychiatric nursing provides specialized care for mental health disorders
- Mental health is essential for overall well-being and is influenced by multiple factors (biological, psychological, social, cultural, economic)
- Determinants of mental health include risk and protective factors that affect illness development and recovery
- Mental health exists on a continuum from wellness to illness; early intervention is crucial
- Cultural and socioeconomic factors affect mental health beliefs, access to care, and treatment outcomes
- Ethical and legal considerations in psychiatric nursing ensure patient rights, confidentiality, and safe practice
- The nursing process (assessment to evaluation) guides individualized mental health care
- Community mental health nursing focuses on prevention, early detection, rehabilitation, and collaboration in community settings

Sample Short Questions

1. Define psychiatric nursing and explain its importance in mental health care.
2. What is the mental health-illness continuum? Why is it important in psychiatric nursing?
3. State the main ethical issues faced by psychiatric nurses in their practice.
4. What roles do psychiatric nurses play in community mental health nursing?

Sample Essay Questions

1. Explain the various determinants of mental health and mental illness and how they influence nursing care.
2. Analyze the impact of cultural and socioeconomic factors on mental health care delivery and nursing interventions.
3. Describe the psychiatric nursing process in detail and explain its significance in patient care.
4. Discuss the importance of community mental health nursing and the role of nurses in promoting mental health in community settings.

Sample Multiple Choice Questions (MCQs) and Sample Best Answers

Which of the following are key components of the psychiatric nursing process?			What is the primary goal of psychiatric nursing?		
T	(a)	Assessment		(a)	To prescribe medication
T	(b)	Diagnosis	✓	(b)	To promote mental health and manage mental illness
F	(c)	Prescription of medications		(c)	To provide surgical care
T	(d)	Planning		(d)	To conduct laboratory tests
F	(e)	Marketing of mental health services			

Suggested Reading

Neeraja, K. P. (2015). *Essentials of mental health nursing* (2nd ed.). Jaypee Brothers Medical Publishers.

Prakash, P. (2022). *Textbook of mental health & psychiatric nursing for BSc students: As per the syllabus of Indian Nursing Council*. CBS Publishers & Distributors Pvt Ltd.

Sreevani R. (2020). *A textbook of mental health (psychiatric) nursing* (4th ed.). Jaypee Brothers Medical Publishers.

Townsend M. C. (2020). *Psychiatric mental health nursing: Concepts of care in evidence-based practice* (10th ed.). F.A. Davis Company.

Chapter 2
Biopsychosocial Theories of Mental Health and Illness

Kulsuma Akter and S. M. Yasir Arafat

Abstract There have been various attempts to explain the causation and treatment approaches in psychiatric disorders. A number of models have been proposed and tested since the inception. The biopsychosocial model is a well-recognized model that underpins key paradigm for advancing mental health research and practice. This chapter outlines the role of the model to understand mental disorders and comprehensive care by integrating biological, psychological, and social factors. Additionally, it highlights how biopsychosocial model addresses health care professional in conceptualizing mental disorders by understanding multidimensional health challenges and patient experiences. It has a substantial clinical implication in understanding mental disorder and clinical decision-making. This chapter also covers model limitations and debates like any other model.

Keywords Biopsychosocial model · Biomedical model · Mental health · Mental disorder · Psychiatric nursing care, and social dimensional effect on a patient's health outcomes

1 Biopsychosocial Model

Biopsychosocial concept was first coined by Roy Grinker in 1954. Later, George Engel, who was introduced biopsychosocial (BPS) model as more scientific in 1977. Bio psychosocial model typically contrasted with biomedical model which deals with core concepts of biological science only. Before insufficient strong empirical or conceptual evidence against biologization of psychiatry, biopsychosocial model was seen as an antidote. In every health care intervention Engel conceptualized

K. Akter
Department of Nursing and Health Science, Jashore University of Science and Technology, Jashore, Bangladesh

S. M. Y. Arafat (✉)
Department of Psychiatry, Bangladesh Specialized Hospital, Dhaka, Bangladesh
e-mail: arafatdmc62@gmail.com

S. M. Y. Arafat and H. Akter (eds.), *Psychiatric Nursing in Bangladesh*, Mental Health Systems and Policy in Low- and Middle-Income Countries,
https://doi.org/10.1007/978-981-95-8501-4_2

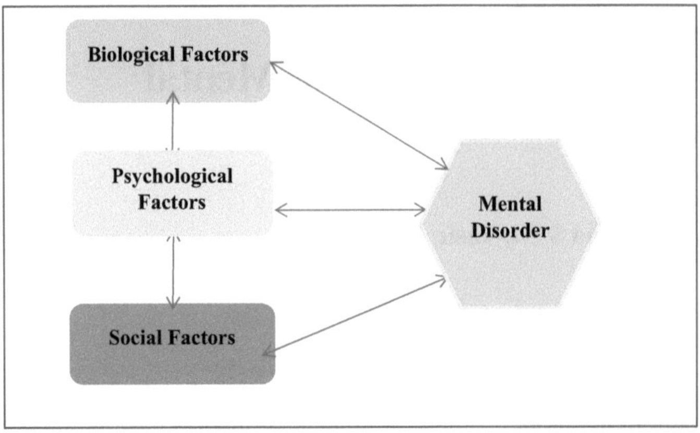

Fig. 1 Biopsychosocial model

the connection among biological, psychological and social domain and claimed this model as 'blueprint for research, a framework for teaching, and a design for action in the real world of health care' (Fig. 1). Although BPS model has several limitations in mental health care, multidimensional approach of BPS model helps understand complex health care issues including schizophrenia, major depressive disorder, depression and substance abuse and explore biological, psychological and social dimensional effect on a patient's health outcomes.

Biological Factors

Biological factors involve physiological and genetic influences on mental health. Family history and genetic predispositions can increase the likelihood of developing mental health problems. Familial, twin, and adoption studies have suggested possible genetic influence on the onset of mental disorders, including schizophrenia, panic disorder, depression, bipolar disorder, anorexia nervosa, alcoholism, Alzheimer's, and obsessive-compulsive disorder. Besides alteration in the number or structure of a chromosome or mutation of a specific or multiple genes, the neurotransmitter hypothesis and endocrine correlation can be seen. Abnormalities in brain chemicals such as dopamine, serotonin, norepinephrine, and acetylcholine are linked to various mental health disorders that are included above.

Psychological Factors

It encompasses the cognitive, emotional, and behavioral aspects that influence mental health. Factors include personality, intelligence, poor parent-child relationship, dysfunctional family systems, verbal abuse, past experience, self-concept and motivation, psychological defenses, and sense of control over oneself.

Example: Childhood maltreatment is considered as a key predisposing factor in developing psychiatric disorder. Several studies have found the consequences of childhood maltreatment including emotional abuse and neglect, verbal abuse, insult, humiliation, threats to abandon or hurt, and statements like "I wish you were never born."

Social Factors

Social factors encompass the environmental and relational contexts that influence mental health. These factors can include lower social economic conditions, congested housing accommodations, inadequate nutrition, poverty, absence of parental care responsible for developing psychiatric disorder such as depression and anxiety.

Example: Postpartum depression (PPD) is a widespread mental health problem in women, with symptoms that can arise within the first 6 weeks after delivery. PPD can also develop for up to a year following delivery. Besides biological, psychological, and social dimensions, some socio-demographic identifiable factors including marital relationship, social support, delivery methods, birth experience, unplanned pregnancy, social economic status, violence, abuse, stress, insufficient or no support from husband, joblessness, or inability to do paid jobs due to pregnancy were significant predictors of post-partum depression.

Interconnections and Implications

Biopsychosocial model addresses not only a broad spectrum of conditions in which incorporating biological, psychological, and social factors relevant to health and disease but also their interactions with one another. A widely applicable example of the biopsychosocial model is pain perception as it includes neurological, psychological, and physiological or structural injury. Treatment approaches that consider all three domains are often the most effective. This may involve medication (to address biological factors), psychotherapy (to target psychological issues), and community support (to strengthen social networks). This model covers the etiology of developing disease, treatment, and also post-onset contributing factors that adversely impact of anticipated outcomes. This model encourages a comprehensive approach to mental health care, promoting not only symptom relief but also overall well-being and resilience.

2 Biological Model

The biological model of mental health and illness, also known as the biomedical/ medical model, posits that mental disorders primarily a result of biological factors. It emphasizes mainly on the role of genetics, neurobiology, and physiological processes in developing of mental health conditions. It is the earliest model explaining disorders. The developments of mental and neuropsychiatric disorders arise from brain biology and their reciprocal interactions with the surrounding environment (Box 1). In practice, diagnoses are grounded on clinical symptoms, rather than on biological or measurable behavioral data.

Common mental disorders like schizophrenia, depression and anxiety have multiple biological mechanisms rather single causal hypotheses. Therefore, advancing biology-based hypotheses requires integrating multimodal evidence including neuroimaging, neurophysiology, digital behavioral measures, and molecular biomarkers.

Box 1: Key Components of the Biological Model

1. **Genetics**—Family and twin studies indicated that genetic predispositions are involved in developing mental disorders like schizophrenia and depression,
2. **Neurotransmitter Systems**—Misbalancing in brain chemicals (e.g., serotonin, dopamine) are linked to mood, behavior, and cognitive disorders.
3. **Brain Structure and Function**—Neuroimaging reveals abnormalities in specific brain areas (e.g., amygdala, prefrontal cortex) associated with various mental disorders.
4. **Physiological Factors**—Chronic illnesses, hormonal changes, and substance abuse impact mental well-being.

Strengths and Limitations of the Biological Model

In medical discourse, biological model grounded on scientific research. This model helps in measuring objectives through test and imaging. This model supports health professionals in administering effective treatment. Besides several strengths this model also has drawbacks. It may contribute to stigma and neglects individual experiences, culture influences and social contexts. In addition, it increasing the tendency of overprescribe psychiatric drugs without considering potential adverse effects.

Implications of the Biological Model in Psychiatric Nursing

Biological model influences psychiatric nursing through focusing on biological factors with incorporating pharmacological treatments, while emphasizing holistic care, patient education about adherence and effects. This model supports in recognizing the genetic, neurochemical, and structural causes of conditions like depression and schizophrenia. This model is also used to explain the biological basis of mental health conditions to reduce stigma and guide healthy lifestyle practices. Nurses implement biological model in evidence based practice and involve in research for improving mental health care.

3 Psychoanalytic Model

Sigmund Freud developed psychoanalytic theory where he divided the mind into three parts as id, ego, and superego. In this theory, he emphasized that the unconscious mind regulates human behavior. He believed that an individual's basic characteristics are established during these early years, which significantly influence one's adaptation styles and personality development in adulthood.

Structure of Personality

Freud proposed the concepts of the id, the ego, and the superego, three major components of human personality that continuously work together and shape individual's behavior.

Id

Freud described id as the earliest and main component of personality that present from birth. By nature, id is self-centered, impulsive but unconscious. All the initiatives of a person towards pleasure and self-satisfaction come from Id. It does not bother about environment. Throughout one's life, id does not develop with age and remains infantile as it operates unconsciously. For example, a child cries loudly because he wants candy immediately, without considering social norms.

Ego

The ego develops from the id, but is modified by the influence of the external world, adjusts to it and responds accordingly. Ego, also called the reality principle, the conscious part of mind that deals with reality.

It acts as a mediator and preserves the balance between external world and id. Example: A hungry baby becomes calm after feeding, indicating the ego's understanding that the need has been fulfilled.

Superego

Superego represents our internal moral standards and values that we learned from family and society. The superego plays an important role in decision-making, judgment, and controls id impulses. It can analyze one's actions, thoughts, and one's feeling of pride and guilt. When a child is rewarded for his good behavior, it enhanced his self-esteem. On the other hand, when a child punished for his misconduct that creates his inner sense of right and wrong.

Levels of Consciousness

Freud explained the development of personality by describing three levels of consciousness: conscious, preconscious, and unconscious. In conscious mind, individuals can easily remember all significant memories and experiences, have a conscious level of personality, and can control goal-oriented behavior. Preconscious mind is the intermediate level between conscious and the unconscious mind. An individual's all memories and knowledge are not in their current awareness, but with attention, they can be recalled. In the unconscious mind, an individual is unable to bring past experiences or memories into conscious awareness. Unconscious material is composed of unpleasant or unnecessary memories that can be retrieved only through therapy, hypnosis, and with substances that alter the awareness and capacity to restructure repressed memories. Unconscious material can emerge in dream and in seemingly incomprehensible behavior.

Psychosexual Stages of Development

Freud believed that personality develops through **five psychosexual stages**, where unresolved conflicts can lead to **fixations** (persistent behaviors linked to earlier stages).

Oral Stage (Birth to 18 months)

During this stage, mainly focus on sucking (e.g., breastfeeding) and exploring object by placing them in mouth. **Example**—Overeating, smoking, or nail-biting in adulthood due to unresolved dependency issues.

Anal Stage (18 months to 3 years)

In anal stage, focus on toilet training and control's this stage is not completed satisfactorily, the child becomes an adult who is either excessively conservation or messy and destructive. **Example**—A child harshly disciplined for toilet training may develop **anal-retentive** (overly neat) or **anal-expulsive** (disorganized) traits in adulthood.

Phallic Stage (3–6 years)

During this stage, awareness of gender roles and attraction to the opposite-sex parent (**Oedipus/Electra complex**) develops. If needs are satisfactorily met, child develops a gender-appropriate identity. **Example**—An unresolved Oedipus complex may lead to relationship difficulties in adulthood.

Latency Stage (6–12 years)

In latency stage, sexual impulses are inactive; children focus on social and intellectual skills. If this stage is successfully completed, becoming adults can deal with various life situations. **Example -** A child develops friendships and academic skills instead of focusing on romantic interests.

Genital Stage (13–20 years)

During this stage, mature sexual interests and romantic relationships develop. In this stage, energy is expanded by establishing psychological dependence from parents and family. **Example**—A healthy adult forming meaningful romantic relationships.

Erikson's theory focused on **psychosocial development rather than psychosexual development**. He divided psychosocial development into eight phases. Every stage of life people faces psychosocial demands that persist into old age (Table 1). To grow, one must overcome each challenge and prepare for the following stage:

Strengths and Limitations of the Psychoanalytic Model

The psychoanalytic model has many advantages. The concepts introduced by Freud affected educators and psychologists, inspired interest in early childhood mental health, and foster the practice of child psychotherapy. Firstly, it provides a framework to explain human behavior in different cycle of life. Secondly, it explores unconscious processes, childhood experiences, and internal conflicts. Thirdly, it focuses on social emotional dimension and helps individuals gain insight into unresolved emotional conflicts. Furthermore, this model emphasizes on the significance of early childhood in shaping personality and behavior. Although it has many benefits, this model also has some limitations. Firstly, it is difficult to test it scientifically. Secondly, adulthood factors are neglected here. Thirdly, it is time-consuming and costly. Therefore, this model is not applicable universally.

Implications of the Psychoanalytic Model in Psychiatric Nursing Care

Psychoanalytic theory helps to consider nurses all aspects of human behavior as well as emphasizes how early childhood experiences have lasting effects on adult

Table 1 Psychosocial development

Stages	Basic conflict	Important events	Outcome
Infancy (birth to 18 months)	Trust vs. mistrust	Feeding	Providing reliable care and affection foster trust; neglect leads mistrust
Early childhood (2–3 years)	Autonomy vs. doubt	Toilet training	Kids gaining confidence by developing control while failure brings doubt
Preschool (3–5 years)	Initiative vs. guilt	Exploration	Children explore power, success builds purpose, and too much power leads to guilt
School age (6–11 years)	Industry vs. inferiority	School	Children need to cope with new social and academic demands. Success leads competence, while failure results inferiority
Adolescence (12–18 years)	Identity vs.confusion	Social relationships	Adolescent shape identity; success brings self-confidence, failure causes confusion
Young adulthood (19 to 40 years)	Intimacy vs.Isolation	Relationships	Intimacy in young adulthood fosters grouth, while failure brings isolation
Middle adulthood (40 to 65 years)	Generativity vs. stagnation	Work and parenthood	Adult focus on contribute to society, gaining fulfillment in success and fiustration in failure
Maturity (65 to death)	Ego integrity vs. despair	Reflection on life	Old-age reflections on life, fulfillment brings wisdom, failure brings regret

personality and psychological growth. Exploring the manifestation of anxiety and identifying maladaptive coping strategies and guiding patient with defense mechanisms are used to problem-solving and emotional regulation. It also helps nurses in understanding insights into how the unconscious mind influences a person's thoughts, emotions, and actions. Early life experience plays a key role in personality development and affects their adult life. Educating parents on their child needs at each psychosexual stage can enhance effective parenting practice.

Defense Mechanisms

Defense mechanisms are individual traits that help people adapt to reality and cope with anxiety. Freud recognized a number of defense mechanisms as the part of ego in the context of biological or psychological integrity. Some of these defense mechanisms are more adaptive (enhance integration with ego) and others are maladaptive (disintegrate with ego). Adaptive defense mechanisms are used to remove unacceptable impulses from conscious awareness to relieve mild to moderate anxiety. The major ego defense mechanisms are discussed in Table 2.

Table 2 Ego defense mechanisms

Defense Mechanisms	Examples
Compensation is the emphasis on a perceived desire for concealing a real weakness	A handicapped student who is unable to study in civil engineering program, compensates by becoming a great English scholar.
Denial is the refusal to accept an unpleasant reality	A chain smoker who denies the harmful effects of smoking.
Displacement is transferring one's unacceptable thought to another that is considered as less threatening	A businessman is angry with his client, does not express it, but becomes verbally rough with his assistant.
Identification is adopting the attribute of an admired person	A student who impressed by his mentor, wants to apply similar teaching strategy in his career
Intellectualization is the attempt to avoid unpleasant feeling by using excessive cognition	An undergraduate level first-year student has to stay in a hall away from home. He conceals his homesickness by explaining his new friends and environment of his university
Isolation is the separation of thoughts from the feelings associated with them. It is also called emotional isolation	A student tells his/her parents about his failure in examination without any emotion
Introjection is adopting beliefs and values of another individual into one's ego structure	A child tells his friends on exam day not to cheat as it is not good
Projection is attributing one's unacceptable impulses or thoughts to another person	A student who arrives late to class, explains that he is late because of delay in receiving information of class schedule from his class representative
Rationalization is justifying undesirable thoughts by using excuse.	A smoker says, "I smoke to get rid of my stress"
Reaction formation is the demonstration of behavior that is directly opposed to one's true feelings	A job candidate who desires to become a bureaucrat, hates any other job advertisements
Regression is taking off personality development to an earlier functional level, which helps to cope up with anxiety	A candidate, after failing in a written recruitment examination, starts playing cricket for long periods of time
Repression is the involuntary removal of unpleasant feeling and experiences from one's awareness	An adolescent who cannot remember being injured by gunshot at early age incident in July '24 massacre
Suppression is the voluntary restriction of unpleasant feelings and experiences from one's awareness	After an argument between two friends, one says, "I don't want to talk about that topic now"
Sublimation is the transformation of impulses that are socially unacceptable into more acceptable ones	A person with a tendency to argue becomes a great lawyer
Undoing is the act of symbolically negating an experience that one finds undesirable	A father, after condemning his daughter, fetches new books and her favorite food for her

4 Social Model

The social model of mental health emphasizes the role of social, environmental, and cultural factors in the development, maintenance, and treatment of mental health conditions. The social model suggested that developing mental health issues are not only for the effects of individual pathology but also has significant influence on broader societal contexts. Key components are described in Table 3.

Strengths and Limitations of Social Model

Social model has several benefits. Firstly, the social model promotes preventive strategies by addressing social determinants and improving community resources. Secondly, it encourages individuals and communities to advocate for their rights and access to mental health resources. Furthermore, this model also contributes in promoting culturally sensitive care that respects individuals' diverse backgrounds. Besides some benefits, social model also has some limitations. Biological factors are neglected while focusing on individual social, cultural, and environmental context. This model has a risk of blame because changing society is difficult as well as expensive.

Table 3 Key Components of the Social Model

Component	Description
Social determinants of mental health	Social determinants of mental health cover conditions including socioeconomic status, education, income, employment, housing, food security, childhood adversity, early life adversity, migration, and healthcare access that drive mental health and disparities
Cultural context	Culture influences the perception, experience, and treatment of mental health. Culturally competent care is essential to address individual beliefs and practices
Relationships and social support	Strong social networks and supportive relationships are vital for mental Well-being. Social isolation and relationship breakdowns contribute to mental health issues
Environmental factors	Living conditions, neighborhood environment, safety, and access to recreational facilities impact mental health. Community resources, including mental health services, are crucial for support
Stigma and discrimination	Stigma and discrimination deter individuals from seeking help and worsen conditions. Raising awareness and promoting understanding are key to reducing stigma

Implications of the Social Model in Psychiatric Nursing Care

By applying this model, nurses assess how factors like socioeconomic status, relationships, and housing contribute to mental health care. This model helps nurses to empower patients in decision-making by showing respect for cultural norms and values in care plans and addressing crises such as domestic violence or homelessness and provide immediate support and referrals.

5 Interpersonal Model

The interpersonal model is rooted in the understanding that mental health issues often arise from difficulties in relationships with others. It plays a critical role in promoting mental health. Harry Stack Sullivan, who is familiar as interpersonal theorist, has outlined six stages of development (Table 4). He believed that every individual has to complete these stages of development for building satisfactory relationship with others.

Strengths and Limitations of the Interpersonal Model

Considering the broader social context of mental health, it helps in recognizing the influence of relationships. This model emphasizes healthy relationships to enhance flexibility and coping. It supports interpersonal therapy to improve interpersonal relationship. Research indicates that strong social support contributes to improved mental health outcomes. It neglects individual psychological, biological, and personal factors. This model may not consider the influence of cultural context in shaping cultural dynamics and mental well-being.

Table 4 Stages of development in Sullivan's interpersonal theory

Stages	Major development tasks
Infancy (birth to 18 months)	Relief anxiety through oral gratification of needs
Childhood (18 months to 6 years)	Learning to accept delay if needs not met immediately
Juvenile (18 years to 9 years)	Forming relationship with peers
Preadolescence (9–12 years)	Learning to form friendship with same sex
Early adolescence (12–14 years)	Learning to become independent and forming satisfactory relationship with opposite gender
Late adolescence (14–21 years)	Establishing close and long-lasting relationship with opposite gender

Implications of the Interpersonal Model in Psychiatric Nursing Care

Nurses create a safe, supportive environment, building trust and empathy to resolve interpersonal difficulties.

6 Lazarus's Theory of Emotion

Psychologist Richard Lazarus developed emotion theory and emphasized the cognitive appraisal process in understanding how emotions are elicited and experienced. According to Lazarus, emotions are not just automatic responses to stimuli; they involve a complex interplay of cognitive processes that determine how individuals perceive and react to situations. Components of Lazarus's theory of emotion are presented in Table 5.

Strengths and Limitations of Lazarus's Theory of Emotion

Lazarus's theory acknowledges the complexity of emotions by considering the interplay of cognitive, behavioral, and physiological components. This theory emphasized the importance of cognitive processes in emotional experiences, moving beyond physiological or behavioral explanations. Though Lazarus's theory has many benefits, also has some drawbacks. This theory does not sufficiently address unconscious influences on emotion and behavior, which may affect the appraisal process. Critics argue that the theory focuses too much on cognitive appraisal, neglecting emotional

Table 5 Key Components of Lazarus's Theory of Emotion

Component	Description
Cognitive appraisal	The process of evaluating and interpreting a situation to determine its significance for Well-being
Primary appraisal	The initial evaluation to determine an individual's ability to cope with stress
Secondary appraisal	Evaluation of coping resources, options for action, and potential outcomes to assess ability to manage the situation
Emotions as responses	Emotions are responses to cognitive appraisals; different appraisals lead to different emotional reactions
Emotion regulation	Managing emotions and coping strategies to adjust appraisals and responses, enhancing Well-being and coping
Context and individual differences	Emotions vary based on context, personality, past experiences, and cultural factors that influence appraisals

and physiological processes that also play important roles in emotional experiences. However, this theory may not account for how different individuals can respond differently to the same situation due to factors like mood, personality, and context.

Implications of Lazarus's Theory of Emotion in Psychiatric Nursing Care

Lazarus's theory offers practical insights for improving emotional regulation, coping, and mental health outcomes in psychiatric nursing. Using cognitive behavioral therapy, nurses help patients modify maladaptive appraisals and boost coping confidence. Nurses create a safe space for emotional expression and validation through active listening and help in reframing negative appraisals in conditions like depression and anxiety including emotional support during crises. Nurses empower patients with coping strategies and a holistic approach to care.

7 Crisis Theory

Crises can arise from a variety of stressors, both external and internal, and are common in people's life. By nature, crises can be social, psychological, or biological. They have both positive and negative impact on one's life. Crisis theory examines the nature of crisis, how individual and systems respond to crises and the processes involved in recovery and adaptation.

Crisis intervention is a skilled, time-limited, and goal-oriented therapeutic approach that helps individuals in responding to stress. As a part of predominant workforce within the healthcare systems, professional nurses play pivotal role for people in times of crisis to promote mental health and healthy outcomes. Paradigm of crisis situation is presented in Fig. 2.

Key Components of Crisis Theory

Crisis is a situation that occurs suddenly resulting from a stressful event or perceived threat.

Characteristics

- Usually occurs suddenly.
- Crisis is personal by nature.
- Most crises are acute but not chronic.
- In situation of crisis, coping method fails and raises one's feelings of fear, anger, anxiety, shame, and hopelessness.

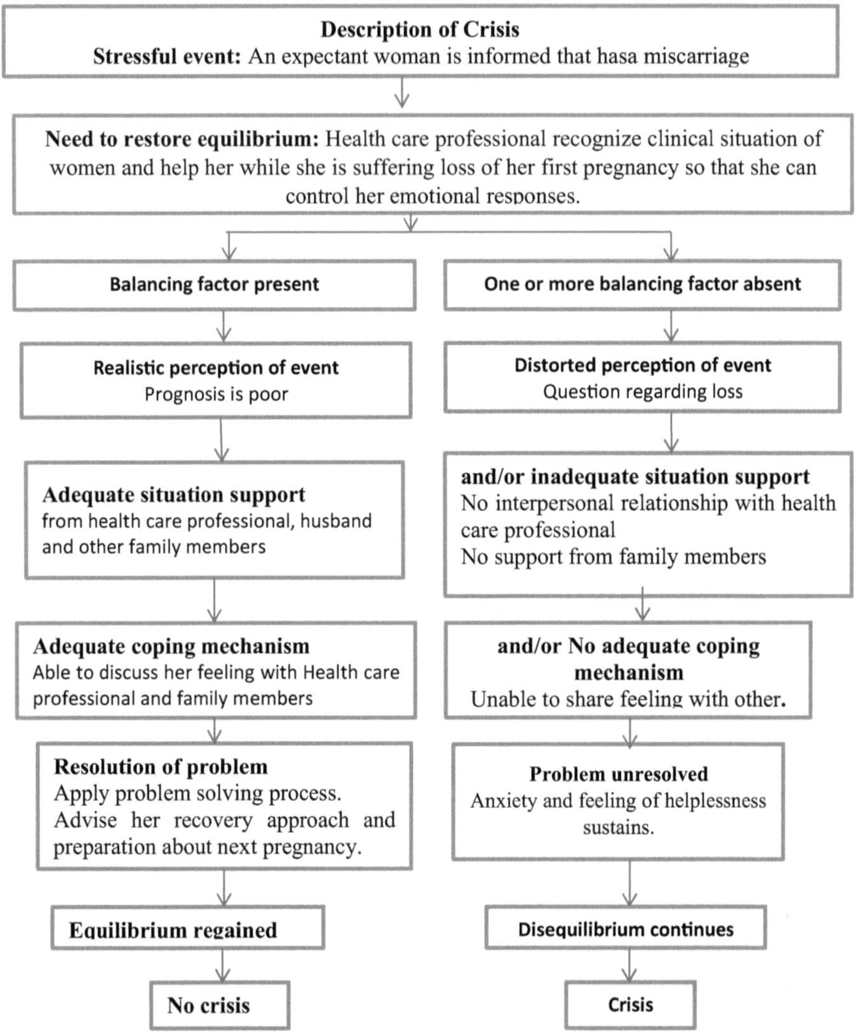

Fig. 2 Paradigm of crisis situation

- If it is not man-made or caused by disaster, most crises last 24–36 hours. It rarely lasts several weeks to years.
- Psychiatric emergency can arise from crises.
- Crisis can offer scope for personal development and post-traumatic growth.

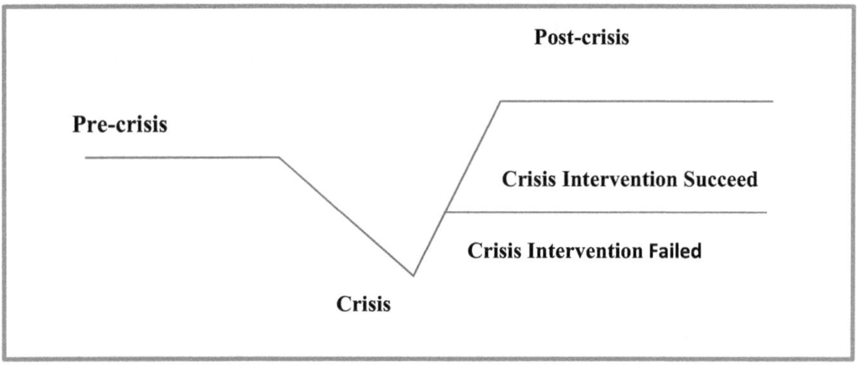

Fig. 3 Phases of crisis

Types of Crises

Crises can be developmental or situational. Sometimes these occur simultaneously in a person's life. For example, an elderly person having worries due to loss of identity after his retiring from job, and at the same time, his family began to neglect care of his needs.

Developmental Crises: Life transitions during adolescence, puberty, parenthood, marriage, and retirement are key times in which developmental crisis onset.

Situational Crises: Unexpected events like accidents, medical or psychiatric illness, child abuse, rape, divorce, loss of hair after chemotherapy, death loved one, and loss of power due to revolution.

Phases of crisis are presented in Fig. 3.

Pre-crisis phase: Vulnerabilities or stressors leading to crisis.

Crisis phase: Emotional and functional disruption.

Post-crisis phase: Recovery, adaptation, and growth.

Strengths and Limitations of Crisis Theory

Crisis theory provides a framework for understanding and addressing crises in various contexts, including mental health, emergency services, and social work. It offers valuable insights for developing effective intervention strategies to support individuals experiencing crises. It enables us to detect psychosocial challenges underlying symptom expression. In addition, it emphasizes the potential for growth and resilience following a crisis, highlighting the importance of recovery processes. Besides benefit, this theory also has some limitations. It has a little application in severely ill psychiatric patient care. It does not properly address dynamic nature of symptom patterns over different periods. The theory may not fully account for cultural differences in understanding and responding to crises. Cultural beliefs and practices can significantly influence crisis experiences and coping mechanisms. Though crisis theory often emphasizes immediate responses to crises, which may overlook the long-term effects of trauma and ongoing support needs.

Implications of Crisis Theory in Psychiatric Nursing Care

Crisis theory helps psychiatric nurses recognize patient's perception, emotional instability, confusion, or anxiety and evaluate the nature of a crisis and its severity for early intervention and manage psychological crises by providing immediate support, promoting resilience, and empowering patients to view challenges as opportunities for growth. Crisis Intervention Strategies help to collaborate with patients to assess the patient's coping strategies and their effectiveness in finding realistic solutions to problems and restore emotional stability. By using this theory, nurses can support in preventing long-term psychological damage (e.g., chronic anxiety or post-traumatic stress disorder) and teaching relaxation techniques by providing immediate support, promoting resilience, and empowering patients to view challenges as opportunities for growth.

Sample Short Answer Questions

1. What is the biopsychosocial model/theory?
2. What is the biological model?
3. Write down the strengths and limitations of the biological model
4. Write down the strengths and limitations of the social model
5. What is the crisis theory?

Sample Essay Questions

1. Discuss the key components of the bio-psychosocial model and how they relate to mental health and illness
2. Write down the importance of the biopsychosocial model/theory in psychiatric nursing care
3. Describe the implications of the biological model in psychiatric nursing care

Sample Multiple Choice (MCQ) and Sample Best Answer Questions

Lazarus's theory of emotion includes-			What does the biological model of mental health primarily focus on?		
T	a)	Cognitive appraisal drives emotion		a)	Environmental factors
F	b)	Emotions bypass thought processes	✓	b)	Genetic and physiological aspects
T	c)	Interpretation impacts stress		c)	Psychological theories
F	d)	Ignores personal experiences		d)	Social influences
T	e)	By Richard Lazarus			

Suggested Reading

Ali, A. (2016). Reflection on Richard Lazarus' emotion and adaptation. *The British Journal of Psychiatry, 209*(5), 399–399. https://doi.org/10.1192/bjp.bp.115.178285

Ball, J. S., Links, P. S., Strike, C., & Boydell, K. M. (2005). 'It's overwhelming … everything seems to be too much:' A theory of crisis for individuals with severe persistent mental illness. *Psychiatric Rehabilitation Journal., 29*(1), 10–17. https://doi.org/10.2975/29.2005.10.17

Baumgardt, J., & Weinmann, S. (2022). Using crisis theory in dealing with severe mental illness–a step toward normalization? *Frontiers in Sociology, 7*, 805604. https://doi.org/10.3389/fsoc.2022.805604

Bolton, D. (2022). Looking forward to a decade of the biopsychosocial model. *BJPsych Bull., 46*(4), 228–232. https://doi.org/10.1192/bjb.2022.34

Bolton, D. (2023). A revitalized biopsychosocial model: Core theory, research paradigms, and clinical implications. *Psychological Medicine, 53*(16), 7504–7511. https://doi.org/10.1017/S0033291723002660

Glowacki, K., Whyte, M., Weinstein, J., Marchand, K., Barbic, D., Scheuermeyer, F., et al. (2022). Exploring how to enhance care and pathways between the emergency department and integrated youth services for young people with mental health and substance use concerns. *BMC Health Services Research, 22*(1), 615. https://doi.org/10.1186/s12913-022-07990-8

Kantor, V., Verginer, L., Glück, T. M., Knefel, M., & Lueger-Schuster, B. (2022). Barriers and facilitators to accessing mental health services after child maltreatment in foster care: An Austrian survivors' perspective. *European Journal of Trauma & Dissociation., 6*(1), 100228. https://doi.org/10.1016/j.ejtd.2021.100228

Kas, M. J. H., Penninx, B. W. J. H., Knudsen, G. M., Cuthbert, B., Falkai, P., Sachs, G. S., et al. (2025). Precision psychiatry roadmap: Towards a biology-informed framework for mental disorders. *Molecular Psychiatry, 30*(8), 3846–3855. https://doi.org/10.1038/s41380-025-03070-5

Kretchy, I. A., Blewuada, E. K., & Debrah, A. B. (2021). A qualitative study exploring community pharmacists' perspectives of child and adolescent mental healthcare. *Scientific African., 13*, e00969. https://doi.org/10.1016/j.sciaf.2021.e00969

Saracho ON. (2023). Theories of child development and their impact on early childhood education and care. *Early Childhood Education Journal, 51*(1), 15–30. https://doi.org/10.1007/s10643-021-01271-5

Solmi, M., Radua, J., Olivola, M., Croce, E., Soardo, L., Salazar De Pablo, G., et al. (2022). Age at onset of mental disorders worldwide: Large-scale meta-analysis of 192 epidemiological studies. *Molecular Psychiatry, 27*(1), 281–295. https://doi.org/10.1038/s41380-021-01161-7

Zifkin, C., Montreuil, M., Beauséjour, M.-È., Picard, S., Gendron-Cloutier, L., & Carnevale, F. A. (2021). An exploration of youth and parents' experiences of child mental health service access. *Archives of Psychiatric Nursing., 35*(5), 549–555. https://doi.org/10.1016/j.apnu.2021.06.006

Chapter 3
Psychotherapeutic Modalities

Rubina Jahan, Hasina Akter, and S. M. Yasir Arafat

Abstract Mental health care draws from a broad spectrum of psychological and biological interventions, each contributing to a holistic understanding of mental health and well-being. This chapter introduces nursing students to the major treatment modalities used in contemporary mental health practice, including psychopharmacology and other biological treatments, psychotherapy approaches, individual and group psychotherapy, family interventions, and psychiatric nursing interventions. These modalities are presented with attention to their theoretical foundations, clinical purposes, and relevance to nursing roles. The chapter emphasizes how nurses engage with these treatments through assessment, therapeutic communication, collaboration with multidisciplinary teams, and ongoing patient support across developmental stages and care settings. By linking theoretical concepts with practical nursing responsibilities, this chapter equips future nurses with a structured and comprehensive understanding of mental health interventions, supporting informed decision-making and effective care.

Keywords Psychotherapy · Therapeutic approaches · Psychiatric nursing · Mental health

R. Jahan
Clinical Psychologist and Chief Executive Officer, The Compassion Collaborative Ltd, Dhaka, Bangladesh

H. Akter
Department of Graduate Nursing, Bangladesh Medical University, Dhaka, Bangladesh

S. M. Y. Arafat (✉)
Department of Psychiatry, Bangladesh Specialized Hospital, Dhaka, Bangladesh
e-mail: arafatdmc62@gmail.com

S. M. Y. Arafat and H. Akter (eds.), *Psychiatric Nursing in Bangladesh*, Mental Health Systems and Policy in Low- and Middle-Income Countries,
https://doi.org/10.1007/978-981-95-8501-4_3

1 Psychopharmacology and Other Biologic Treatments

Psychopharmacology is the study of how drugs affect mood, behavior, and mental processes. It encompasses the use of medications to treat psychiatric disorders and examines the interactions between these medications and the brain. Psychopharmacology and other biological treatments involve the use of medications and biological interventions to manage psychiatric disorders. These approaches are grounded in the understanding that biological factors—such as neurochemistry, genetics, and physiological processes play a crucial role in the development and treatment of mental illnesses.

2 Other Biological Treatments

Psychotropic medications are drugs that affect brain function and are used to treat various mental health conditions. They are classified based on their mechanism of action and therapeutic effects (Table 1, Fig. 1).

Anti-psychotics

Antipsychotic drugs (also called neuroleptics) are used to manage symptoms of psychosis, including hallucinations, delusions, and thought disorders, commonly seen in schizophrenia and other psychotic disorders.

Types:

- Typical (First-Generation)—e.g., Haloperidol, Chlorpromazine, Trifluperazine.
- Atypical (Second-Generation)—e.g., Olanzapine, Risperidone, Clozapine, Aripiprazole, Cariprazine, Lurasidone.

Indications:

- Schizophrenia.
- Bipolar disorder.
- Delusional disorders.
- Severe agitation and aggression.

Contraindications:

- Hypersensitivity to the drug.
- Severe cardiac conditions (QT prolongation).
- Liver or kidney impairment.
- Parkinson's disease (for some typical antipsychotics).

Table 1 Common classes of psychotropic medications

Class	Groups	Brand	Indication
Antipsychotics	First-generation (typical/conventional)	Haloperidol (Halopid)	Schizophrenia Bipolar disorder Psychotic disorders Depression
	Second-generation (atypical/newer)	Risperidone (Residon)	
		Olanzapine (Olanap)	
		Quetiapine (quiet)	
Antidepressants	SSRIs	Fluoxetine (Prolert)	Depression Anxiety disorders Panic disorder OCD PTSD GAD Neuropathic pain
		Sertraline (repose)	
	SNRIs	Venlafaxine (Venlax)	
	TCAs	Amitriptyline (Amilin)	
	MAOIs	Phenelzine	
Mood stabilizers	Lithium	Lithium carbonate (Lithosun)	Bipolar disorder Seizure disorder
	Anticonvulsants	Valproic acid (Valex)	
		Lamotrigine (Lamogin)	
Anxiolytics/sedatives	Benzodiazepines	Diazepam (Sedil)	Anxiety Muscle spasms Seizures Insomnia Agitation
		Lorazepam (Lozicum)	
	Non-benzodiazepine hypnotics	Zolpidem	
Stimulants	Modafinil	Armoda	ADHD Narcolepsy
	Methylphenidate	Alaradate	
Cognitive enhancers	Acetylcholinesterase inhibitors	Donepezil (Ameloss)	Alzheimer's disease Other dementia
	NMDA receptor antagonists	Memantine (Dementa)	

SSRI- Selective serotonin reuptake inhibitor, SNRI- Serotonin-Norepinephrine Reuptake Inhibitor, TCA- Tricyclic Antidepressants, MAOI- Monoamine oxidase inhibitor, NMDA- N-methyl-D-aspartate, OCD- Obsessive-compulsive disorder, PTSD- Post-traumatic stress disorder, GAD-Generalized Anxiety Disorder, ADHD- Attention deficit hyperactivity disorder.

Side Effects:

- Extrapyramidal symptoms (EPS)—dystonia, akathisia, tardive dyskinesia.
- Sedation.
- Weight gain (more common in atypical antipsychotics).
- Metabolic syndrome (diabetes, hyperlipidemia).

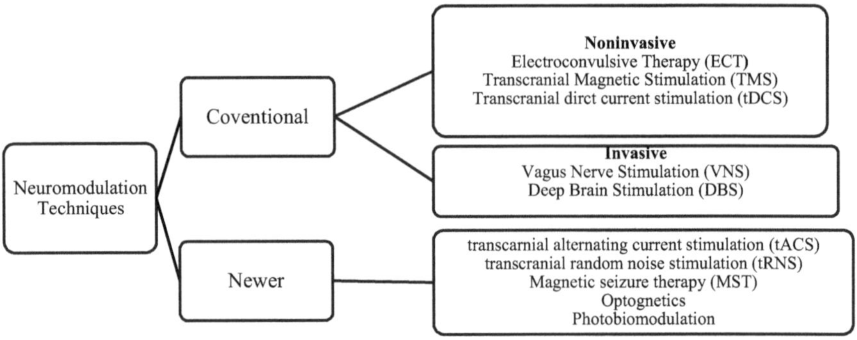

Fig. 1 Neuromodulation techniques

- Neuroleptic malignant syndrome (NMS)—a life-threatening reaction.

Nurse's Role:

- Monitor for EPS and metabolic side effects.
- Educate the patient on adherence and side effects (Box 1).
- Assess for signs of NMS (fever, muscle rigidity).
- Monitor weight, blood glucose, and lipid profile.

Antidepressants

Antidepressants are used to treat depressive disorders by increasing neurotransmitters like serotonin, norepinephrine, and dopamine.

Classes:

- Selective Serotonin Reuptake Inhibitors (SSRIs)—e.g., Fluoxetine, Sertraline, Escitalopram, Vortioxetine, Vilazodone, Paroxetine.
- Serotonin-Norepinephrine Reuptake Inhibitors (SNRIs)—e.g., Venlafaxine, Duloxetine, Des-venlafaxine, Milnacipran, Levomilnacipran.
- Tricyclic Antidepressants (TCAs)—e.g., Amitriptyline, Imipramine, Clomipramine.
- Monoamine Oxidase Inhibitors (MAOIs)—e.g., Phenelzine, Tranylcypromine.
- Atypical Antidepressants—e.g., Bupropion, Mirtazapine.

Indications:

- Major depressive disorder (MDD).
- Anxiety disorders—Generalized Anxiety Disorder (GAD), Post-traumatic stress disorder (PTSD), Panic Disorder, Phobic Disorders.
- Obsessive-compulsive disorder (OCD).
- Chronic pain (TCAs and SNRIs).

Contraindications:

- MAOIs require dietary restrictions (avoid tyramine-rich foods).
- History of seizures (Bupropion).
- Recent use of MAOIs (risk of serotonin syndrome).

Side Effects:

- SSRIs: Nausea, insomnia, sexual dysfunction.
- SNRIs: Hypertension, dizziness.
- TCAs: Sedation, dry mouth, orthostatic hypotension.
- MAOIs: Hypertensive crisis if taken with tyramine-rich foods.

Nurse's Role:

- Educate about delayed onset (takes 2–4 weeks for effects).
- Monitor for suicidal ideation (especially in adolescents).
- Avoid abrupt discontinuation (withdrawal symptoms).
- Monitor blood pressure (especially with SNRIs and MAOIs).

Mood Stabilizers

Mood stabilizers are used to manage mood fluctuations, particularly in bipolar disorder.

Types:

- Lithium.
- Anticonvulsants—e.g., Valproate, Carbamazepine, Lamotrigine.

Indications:

- Bipolar disorder.
- Schizoaffective disorder.
- Impulse control disorders.
- MDD.

Contraindications:

- Kidney disease (for Lithium).
- Pregnancy (Valproate, Carbamazepine, Lithium).
- Liver disease (Valproate).

Side Effects:

- Lithium: Tremors, polyuria, hypothyroidism, lithium toxicity.
- Valproate: Weight gain, liver dysfunction, hair loss.
- Carbamazepine: Blood dyscrasias, dizziness.

Nurse's Role:

- Monitor lithium levels (therapeutic range: 0.6–1.2 mEq/L).
- Encourage fluid intake to prevent toxicity.
- Monitor liver function tests (for Valproate).
- Educate on signs of toxicity (vomiting, diarrhea, tremors).

Anxiolytics

These medications help reduce excessive anxiety and agitation.

Types:

- Benzodiazepines—e.g., Diazepam, Lorazepam, Alprazolam.
- Non-Benzodiazepines—e.g., Buspirone, Hydroxyzine.

Indications:

- GAD.
- Panic disorder.
- Insomnia (short-term).
- Seizures (Benzodiazepines).

Contraindications:

- Respiratory depression (e.g., COPD, sleep apnea)
- Pregnancy (Benzodiazepines)

Side Effects:

- Drowsiness, dizziness
- Cognitive impairment
- Dependence and withdrawal symptoms

Nurse's Role:

- Educate on short-term use to prevent dependence
- Avoid alcohol and CNS depressants
- Monitor for withdrawal symptoms
- Encourage non-pharmacological interventions (e.g., CBT)

Psychostimulants

Stimulants enhance dopamine and norepinephrine activity to improve focus and alertness

Types:

- Methylphenidate—e.g., Alaradate

- Modafinil—e.g., Armoda (not available in Bangladesh)

Indications:

- ADHD
- Narcolepsy

Contraindications:

- Cardiac disease (risk of arrhythmias)
- History of substance abuse
- Anxiety disorders (may worsen symptoms)

Side Effects:

- Insomnia, weight loss
- Increased heart rate and blood pressure
- Irritability and agitation

Nurse's Role:

- Monitor growth in children (height, weight)
- Educate on morning administration to prevent insomnia
- Monitor for signs of misuse or dependence

Sedative-Hypnotics

These medications promote sleep and relaxation

Types:

- Benzodiazepines—e.g., Clonazepam, Midazolam
- Non-Benzodiazepines (Z-drugs)—e.g., Zolpidem, Eszopiclone, Zaleplone (not available in Bangladesh)
- Melatonin Agonists—e.g., Ramelteon, Melatonin (Tab. Filfresh)

Indications:

- Insomnia
- Anxiety (short-term use)

Contraindications:

- History of substance abuse
- Respiratory disorders
- Pregnancy (Benzodiazepines)

Side Effects:

- Drowsiness, dizziness
- Sleepwalking (Z-drugs)
- Tolerance and dependence

Nurse's Role:

- Educate on short-term use to avoid dependence
- Monitor for daytime sedation
- Encourage good sleep hygiene

Extrapyramidal Side Effects (EPSE) of Antipsychotics.

Extrapyramidal symptoms are motor side effects caused by dopamine blockade in the basal ganglia (meso-limbic pathway), primarily with first-generation (typical) antipsychotics.

3 Types of EPS

Dystonia:

- Acute muscle spasms or abnormal postures, often affect the neck (torticollis), face, tongue, or back

Akathisia:

- A feeling of inner restlessness with an inability to stay still.
- Patients may pace or tap their feet

Parkinsonism:

- Symptoms mimic Parkinson's disease and include:
  - Bradykinesia (slowed movement)
  - Rigidity (stiff muscles)
  - Tremors (especially at rest)
  - Mask-like facial expression

Tardive Dyskinesia (TD):

- Involuntary, repetitive movements such as grimacing, lip-smacking, or tongue protrusion
- Often occurs with long-term use

Box 1: Common Reasons for Noncompliance (Not Taking Medication as Prescribed)

1. **Lack of Insight:** Patients may not recognize they are ill and see no need for medication
2. **Side Effects:** Unpleasant effects like weight gain, sedation, or movement disorders discourage adherence
3. **Stigma:** Fear of being labeled or judged for taking psychiatric medication
4. **Poor Communication:** Insufficient explanation about medication benefits and side effects
5. **Cognitive Barriers:** Forgetfulness or apathy due to cognitive impairment or depression
6. **Financial Issues:** High cost or difficulty accessing medication
7. **Substance Use:** Co-occurring drug or alcohol abuse interferes with adherence
8. **Delayed Effects:** Frustration with slow onset of therapeutic benefits
9. **Cultural/Religious Beliefs:** Preference for traditional remedies or spiritual healing
10. **Complex Regimens:** Difficult schedules or multiple medications

4 Electroconvulsive Therapy (ECT)

It is a medical treatment in which a small, controlled electric current is passed through the brain, intentionally triggering a brief seizure. It is performed under general anesthesia and with muscle relaxants. ECT is primarily used to treat severe mental health disorders when other treatments have been ineffective (Table 2).

Table 2 Indications and contraindications of electroconvulsive therapy

Indications	Contraindications
Severe depression—Treatment-resistant, suicidal ideation, refusal to eat/drink	**Absolute: Increased intracranial pressure (ICP)**—Risk of worsening brain swelling
Bipolar disorder—Severe manic or depressive episodes	**Relative:** Recent **myocardial infarction** (heart attack)
Schizophrenia—Catatonia, severe psychosis, treatment-resistant cases	**Uncontrolled hypertension**
Acute suicidal behavior—Immediate intervention needed	**Aneurysms** (cerebral or aortic)
Catatonia—Severe stupor or mutism	**Severe cardiovascular disease**
Neuroleptic malignant syndrome (NMS)—Non-responsive to other treatments	**Severe osteoporosis**
Severe psychosis—With aggression, agitation, or food refusal	**Retinal detachment**
	High-risk pregnancy

5 Complications of ECT.

While ECT is considered safe and effective, complications may occur. Nurses play an important role during ECT (Table 3). These can be categorized into **immediate, short-term, and long-term** complications:

1. Immediate Complications (During or right after the procedure)

- **Headache**: Common due to seizure activity or anesthesia
- **Nausea and Vomiting**: Post-anesthetic side effect
- **Muscle Pain or Soreness**: Resulting from the use of muscle relaxants or seizure activity
- **Transient Confusion**: Patients may experience disorientation post-ECT, lasting for minutes to hours
- Cardiovascular Effects:
- Transient tachycardia (increased heart rate)
- Hypertension (elevated blood pressure)
- Arrhythmias (irregular heart rhythms)
- Rarely, myocardial infarction or cardiac arrest occurs in patients with underlying heart disease
- **Aspiration:** If pre-procedure fasting is not adequate
- **Fractures/Dislocations:** Rare due to modern use of muscle relaxants

2. Short-Term Complications.

- **Memory Loss (Retrograde Amnesia):** Difficulty recalling events just before or after treatment. Typically resolves within days to weeks
- **Anterograde Amnesia:** Temporary difficulty in forming new memories after ECT
- **Prolonged Seizures:** Seizure lasting more than the intended duration
- **Dental or Oral Injuries:** From biting down during the procedure (rare due to mouth guards)

3. Long-Term Complications.

- **Persistent Memory Loss:** Some patients may experience longer lasting retrograde amnesia, especially for autobiographical events. This is more common with bilateral ECT
- **Cognitive Impairment**: Rare but may occur in patients receiving high numbers of ECT sessions
- **Mood Fluctuations:** Temporary changes in mood, such as irritability or agitation

Table 3 Role of psychiatric nurse in ECT

Phase	Nursing responsibilities
Pre-ECT (before the procedure)	**obtain informed consent**: Ensure the patient or legal guardian signs the consent form after explaining the procedure, benefits, risks, and alternatives
	physical and mental assessment: Assess baseline vital signs (BP, HR, RR, SpO_2, temperature), mental status, and neurological functioning
	pre-ECT investigations: Ensure completion of laboratory tests (CBC, electrolytes), ECG, and chest X-ray (if needed)
	NPO status: Maintain nothing by mouth (NPO) for at least 6–8 hours before ECT to prevent aspiration
	medication management: Administer pre-medications as prescribed (e.g., atropine or glycopyrrolate to reduce secretions). Hold medications that may interfere with seizure threshold (e.g., benzodiazepines)
	patient preparation: Remove dentures, jewelry, contact lenses, and hearing aids. Ensure the patient has emptied their bladder before the procedure
	emotional support: Reduce anxiety by reassuring the patient, providing clear explanations, and addressing concerns
	intravenous access: Ensure a patent IV line for anesthesia and muscle relaxant administration
During ECT (procedure phase)	**assist in positioning**: Help position the patient supine on the ECT table
	monitor vital signs: Continuously observe heart rate, blood pressure, and oxygen saturation
	support anesthesia administration: Assist in the administration of short-acting anesthetics (e.g., methohexital, propofol) and muscle relaxants (e.g., succinylcholine)
	provide oxygen support: Ensure oxygenation via a face mask before and after seizure induction
	ensure safety: Apply a mouth guard to prevent tongue biting. Maintain airway patency and be prepared for emergency resuscitation if needed
	observe seizure activity: Monitor the duration and type of seizure induced (optimal seizure duration is 15–60 seconds). Report any abnormalities
Post-ECT (recovery phase)	**monitor recovery**: Observe the patient in the post-anesthesia care unit (PACU) until full consciousness is regained
	check vital signs: Assess BP, HR, RR, SpO_2, and temperature frequently. Watch for complications like hypotension, bradycardia, or respiratory distress
	assess cognitive function: Monitor for confusion, memory loss, or disorientation, and provide gentle reorientation
	manage side effects: Offer pain relief for headaches, encourage rest, and provide fluids to prevent dehydration
	ensure safety: Keep the patient under supervision until they are fully alert to prevent falls or injuries

(continued)

Table 3 (continued)

Phase	Nursing responsibilities
	emotional reassurance: Support the patient and family members in coping with temporary memory disturbances and other post-ECT effects
	document the procedure: Record vital signs, duration of seizure, medications given, patient response, and any adverse reactions

6 Psychotherapy: Individual and Group

Psychotherapy is a therapeutic approach aimed at helping individuals and groups understand and manage their thoughts, feelings, and behaviors. It encompasses various modalities and techniques tailored to meet the unique needs of clients.

Definition of Psychotherapy

Psychotherapy, often referred to as talk therapy, is a structured, evidence-based psychological intervention designed to improve mental health and emotional well-being. It employs evidence-based interventions to help individuals understand and modify patterns of thoughts, emotions, and behaviors that contribute to psychological distress or impaired functioning. Two definitions are widely cited in the global literature.

The American Psychological Association (APA) defines psychotherapy as: "the informed and intentional application of clinical methods and interpersonal stances derived from established psychological principles for the purpose of assisting people to modify their behaviors, cognitions, emotions, and/or other personal characteristics in directions that the participants deem desirable".

Similarly, the World Health Organization (WHO) describes it as: "a psychological treatment in which a trained therapist uses evidence-based psychological techniques to help people overcome problems such as mental disorders, emotional difficulties or stress-related problems by improving coping strategies and enhancing functioning".

In essence, psychotherapy is a planned and collaborative process, delivered by trained professionals using well-established psychological theories and empirically validated techniques. Its primary goals are to reduce psychological distress, enhance coping strategies, and promote personal growth and adaptive functioning. These principles apply across different age groups, mental health conditions, and relational contexts, highlighting psychotherapy's versatility as a treatment modality (Box 2, 3).

7 Classification of Psychotherapy

A) The Psychodynamic Approach:

The psychodynamic approach is a broad theoretical framework that includes various therapeutic models rooted in the work of Sigmund Freud, the founder of Psychoanalysis. While these models differ in their specific techniques and areas of focus, they share core assumptions such as unconscious processes influence thoughts and behavior, early childhood experiences shape personality patterns, internalized relationships form the foundation of personality structure, and bringing unconscious material into awareness promotes psychological change. Within this tradition, classical psychoanalysis and Adlerian therapy represent two important but distinctly different approaches.

Psychoanalysis

Classical psychoanalysis is the original and most intensive form of psychodynamic treatment, developed by Sigmund Freud in the late nineteenth century. The method focuses on uncovering unconscious conflicts through specific techniques, including *free association* (verbalizing thoughts without censorship), *dream analysis* (interpreting dreams to access unconscious material), and *analysis of transference* (examining how clients relate to the therapist in ways that reflect earlier relationships). The treatment process of psychoanalysis is intensive, which typically requires multiple sessions per week over several years. It aims for deep personality change rather than simply reducing symptoms.

Modern psychodynamic therapies derive from this model, such as *brief psychodynamic therapy* and time-limited dynamic psychotherapy (TLDP), which generally use shorter, more focused treatment formats suited to contemporary clinical settings.

B) Existential and Relationship-Oriented Therapies

Existential, person-centered, and Gestalt approaches constitute a cluster of existential and relationship-oriented therapies united by shared philosophical commitments and therapeutic priorities. These approaches emphasize personal meaning-making, authentic interpersonal connection, and the therapeutic relationship as a primary agent of change. Although each approach reflects distinct theoretical origins and employs different technical interventions, they converge on a fundamental principle: psychological growth emerges through enhanced self-awareness and genuine engagement with lived experience.

Existential Therapy

Existential therapy addresses the fundamental concerns inherent in human existence, including freedom and its accompanying responsibility, the reality of mortality, the experience of isolation, and the continuous search for meaning. From this perspective, psychological distress is understood not as pathology but as a natural human response to these universal existential challenges. The therapeutic process involves helping clients directly confront these existential realities, accept personal responsibility for their choices, and actively construct meaning and purpose in their lives. Rather than focusing primarily on symptom reduction, existential therapy seeks to promote authenticity and deepen clients' understanding of their core values and the choices that flow from them.

Person-Centered Therapy

Person-centered therapy, developed by Carl Rogers, positions the therapeutic relationship itself as the central mechanism of psychological healing. The approach rests on the assumption that individuals possess an inherent tendency toward growth and self-actualization that emerges naturally when facilitative environmental conditions are present. The therapist's role is to provide three core conditions: *unconditional positive regard* (non-judgmental acceptance), *empathy* (deep understanding of the client's subjective experience), and *genuineness* (authentic presence). These conditions create a safe relational space in which clients can freely explore their feelings and experiences. The therapist does not direct the therapeutic process or offer expert guidance; instead, the therapist trusts and supports the client's own capacity to discover solutions and achieve personal growth.

Gestalt Therapy

Gestalt therapy emphasizes heightened awareness of present-moment experience and the integration of thoughts, emotions, and bodily sensations into a unified whole. Clients are encouraged to assume responsibility for their experiences and to address unfinished business from the past that continues to influence current functioning. The approach employs experiential techniques such as role-play, empty-chair dialogue, and other creative experiments that bring conflicts and feelings into immediate awareness. Through these methods, clients learn to recognize habitual patterns, express emotions more fully and directly, and develop a more coherent and integrated sense of self.

C) **Cognitive Behavioral Approaches**

Cognitive behavioral movement demonstrated that learning principles initially derived from experimental animal research could be effectively applied to modify human behavior. As the field matured, clinicians increasingly recognized that cognitive processes, particularly thoughts and beliefs, play a central role in emotional distress and behavioral patterns. This recognition led to the systematic integration of cognitive and behavioral principles into a family of therapies that address both maladaptive cognition and problematic behavior. These approaches are characterized by their structured format, time-limited duration, and strong empirical foundation. They currently represent among the most extensively researched and widely implemented forms of psychotherapy. Three major therapeutic modalities within this tradition are Behavior Therapy, Cognitive Behavioral Therapy (CBT), and Rational Emotive Behavior Therapy (REBT).

Behavior Therapy

Behavior therapy is grounded in principles of classical and operant conditioning and focuses exclusively on observable behaviors rather than unconscious processes or internal cognitive states. Core techniques include *systematic desensitization* (gradual exposure paired with relaxation), *exposure therapy* (direct confrontation with feared stimuli), and *behavior modification* (systematic reinforcement strategies). These methods aim to reduce maladaptive behavioral responses while strengthening more adaptive patterns. Behavior therapy has demonstrated efficacy in the treatment of specific phobias, obsessive-compulsive disorder, and various anxiety-related conditions.

Cognitive Behavioral Therapy (CBT)

CBT emerged as a conceptual and technical extension of behavior therapy. It incorporates the fundamental premise that cognitive processes directly influence emotional responses and behavioral outcomes. The approach seeks to identify and modify dysfunctional thought patterns while simultaneously promoting behavioral change. Core techniques of CBT include *cognitive restructuring* (identifying and challenging distorted thinking), *behavioral experiments* (testing beliefs through real-world actions), *exposure-based interventions,* and *skills training* (developing specific coping competencies). This structured, goal-directed approach has accumulated extensive empirical support across a broad range of psychological disorders, including major depressive disorder, generalized anxiety disorder, post-traumatic stress disorder, panic disorder, and numerous other conditions.

Rational Emotive Behavior Therapy (REBT)

REBT is predicated on the principle that *irrational beliefs* rather than external events themselves constitute the primary source of emotional distress and dysfunctional behavior. The approach employs the *ABC model* as its central organizing framework, which means *Activating events (A)* trigger *Beliefs (B),* which in turn produce emotional and behavioral *Consequences (C).* Therapists work collaboratively with clients to identify irrational beliefs, vigorously challenge their logical and empirical basis, and replace them with more rational and adaptive cognitions. REBT is characterized by active, directive therapeutic techniques and has demonstrated effectiveness for conditions including chronic anxiety, anger dysregulation, and persistent self-defeating thought patterns.

D) **Third Wave Therapies**

Third-wave therapies are also termed third-generation cognitive-behavioral therapies. It represents approaches that emerged following traditional behavior therapy (the first wave) and cognitive behavior therapy (the second wave). Third-wave approaches, which began emerging in the 1990s, retain the empirical foundation of earlier CBT models while introducing significant conceptual shifts. Rather than focusing primarily on changing the content of thoughts or eliminating problematic behaviors, third-wave therapies emphasize acceptance, mindfulness, contextual factors, values-based action, and the therapeutic relationship. These approaches encourage clients to change their relationship with internal experiences (thoughts, emotions, sensations) rather than attempting to directly modify or eliminate them. Prominent third-wave modalities include *Acceptance and Commitment Therapy (ACT), Dialectical Behavior Therapy (DBT), Mindfulness-Based Cognitive Therapy (MBCT), and Mindfulness-Based Stress Reduction (MBSR).*

Acceptance and Commitment Therapy (ACT)

Acceptance and Commitment Therapy, developed by **Steven Hayes** and colleagues was formalized in the 1990s. ACT does not aim to reduce or eliminate difficult thoughts and feelings; instead, it teaches clients to accept these experiences while committing to behavior aligned with personal values. The approach employs six core processes: *acceptance, cognitive diffusion* (changing one's relationship with thoughts), *contact with the present moment, self-as-context* (observing self), *values clarification, and committed action.* Through experiential exercises and metaphors, ACT helps clients develop psychological flexibility. It refers to the ability to stay present and take valued action even in the presence of uncomfortable internal experiences. The approach has demonstrated efficacy across diverse conditions, including anxiety, depression, chronic pain, and substance use disorders.

Dialectical Behavior Therapy (DBT)

Dialectical Behavior Therapy was developed by Marsha Linehan in the late 1980s. It was originally developed to treat individuals with borderline personality disorder and chronic suicidal behavior. DBT integrates cognitive-behavioral techniques. The term "dialectical" refers to the balance between acceptance and change, which aims to validate clients' experiences while simultaneously working toward behavioral modification. DBT consists of four skill modules: *mindfulness* (present-moment awareness), *distress tolerance* (crisis survival strategies), *emotion regulation* (understanding and managing emotions), *and interpersonal effectiveness* (communicating needs and maintaining relationships). Treatment typically includes individual therapy, skills training groups, phone coaching, and therapist consultation teams. DBT has expanded beyond its original application and is now used effectively for eating disorders, substance use, depression, and other conditions involving emotion dysregulation.

Mindfulness-Based Cognitive Therapy (MBCT)

Mindfulness-Based Cognitive Therapy was developed by Zindel Segal, Mark Williams, and John Teasdale in the 1990s specifically to prevent relapse in recurrent depression. MBCT integrates mindfulness meditation practices with elements of cognitive therapy, teaching clients to recognize and disengage from negative thinking patterns that can trigger depressive episodes. The approach is typically delivered in an eight-week group format, with participants learning to observe thoughts and feelings without judgment or automatic reaction. Rather than challenging the content of negative thoughts (as in traditional CBT), MBCT teaches clients to change their relationship with these thoughts by recognizing them as mental events rather than facts. This metacognitive awareness helps prevent the escalation of negative thought patterns into full depressive relapse. Research has demonstrated that MBCT significantly reduces relapse rates in individuals with a history of recurrent depression.

Mindfulness-Based Stress Reduction (MBSR)

Mindfulness-Based Stress Reduction was developed by Jon Kabat Zinn at the University of Massachusetts Medical Center in 1979. MBSR is a structured eight-week group program that teaches mindfulness meditation practices to help individuals cope with stress, pain, and illness. The program includes formal practices such as body scan meditation, sitting meditation, and gentle yoga, as well as informal mindfulness practices integrated into daily life. Unlike traditional psychotherapy, MBSR does not focus on specific psychological disorders but rather cultivates moment-to-moment awareness and acceptance of experience. Originally developed for chronic pain management, MBSR has been adapted for diverse populations and conditions, with research supporting its effectiveness for stress reduction, anxiety, depression, chronic pain, and overall well-being.

E) **Postmodern Approaches in Psychotherapy**

Postmodern approaches in psychotherapy emerged during the late twentieth century as a conceptual shift away from traditional models. In contrast to the typical emphasis on objective diagnosis, universal truths, and linear causal explanations for psychological problems, postmodern therapies focus on the co-construction of meaning, the influence of social context, and the centrality of client narratives. These approaches understand reality as subjective and shaped by relationships, culture, and language rather than as fixed and objectively knowable conditions. Three prominent post-modern approaches are *Solution-Focused Brief Therapy (SFBT), Narrative Therapy, and Family Systems Therapy.*

While postmodern therapies are effective for individual clients, their focus on collaboration, meaning-making, and social context makes them particularly valuable in relational settings. Couples and families can benefit from solution-focused strategies, narrative re-authoring, and systemic interventions that promote healthier communication and adaptive relational patterns.

Box 2: Indications for Psychotherapy

Mental Health Disorders—Depression, anxiety, bipolar disorder, schizophrenia (adjunct therapy)

Trauma & Stress-Related Conditions—Acute Stress Disorder, Post Traumatic Stress Disorder, and adjustment disorders

Substance Use Disorders—Alcohol/drug addiction, behavioral addictions (e.g., gambling)

Personality Disorders—Borderline personality disorder (BPD), narcissistic personality disorder

Behavioral & Emotional Problems—Anger management, emotional regulation, impulse control disorders

Relationship & Family Issues—Marital conflicts, parent-child relationship problems

Chronic Illness & Pain Management—Coping with cancer, diabetes, chronic pain

Workplace & Academic Stress—Job-related stress, school anxiety, performance issues

Box 3: Goals of Psychotherapy

1. Improve Emotional Well-Being: Manage emotions like anxiety, anger, and sadness
2. Enhance Self-Awareness: Gain insight into thoughts, feelings, and behaviors
3. Develop Coping Strategies: Build skills to handle stress and challenges
4. Modify Maladaptive Patterns: Change negative thoughts and behaviors
5. Strengthen Relationships: Improve communication and interpersonal skills
6. Boost Resilience and Self-Esteem: Enhance confidence and problem-solving
7. Reduce Mental Health Symptoms: Alleviate depression, anxiety, and psychosis
8. Encourage Personal Growth: Promote self-acceptance and fulfillment
9. Prevent Relapse: Maintain progress and prevent recurrence
10. Enhance Quality of Life: Improve emotional, social, and occupational well-being

8 Individual Psychotherapy

Definition of Individual Psychotherapy

Individual psychotherapy involves one-on-one sessions between a therapist and a client. This approach provides a safe and confidential space for individuals to explore personal issues, gain insights, and develop coping strategies (Box 4, Table 4).

Components of Individual Therapy

Individual therapy is a one-on-one session between a therapist and a client, focusing on personal issues and mental health concerns. The key components include:

Table 4 Benefits and limitations of individual therapy

Benefits	Limitations
Personalized treatment plan: Tailored interventions based on the individual's unique needs and circumstances	Cost and accessibility: Can be expensive and may not be accessible to everyone
Confidentiality: A safe space for clients to express their thoughts and feelings without judgment	Dependence on the therapist—Clients may become overly reliant on their therapist for support and guidance
Depth of exploration: Allows for deeper exploration of personal issues and emotional experiences	Limited perspective—Therapy may lack the broader perspectives that group or family therapy could offer

A. Therapeutic Relationship

- Establishing trust and rapport between the therapist and client.
- Providing a safe and non-judgmental space for self-expression.

B. Assessment and Diagnosis

- Understanding the client's history, symptoms, and concerns.
- Conducting psychological assessments, if necessary.

C. Goal Setting

- Defining short-term and long-term therapy goals.
- Collaborating with the client on treatment planning.

D. Intervention Techniques

- Identifying and modifying negative thoughts (e.g., CBT).
- Encouraging positive behaviors (e.g., Exposure Therapy).
- Exploring unconscious conflicts (e.g., Psychoanalysis).
- Teaching stress-reduction strategies (e.g., Mindfulness and Relaxation).

E. Monitoring Progress

- Evaluating the effectiveness of therapy.
- Modifying treatment plans based on client response.

F. Termination and Follow-Up

- Preparing the client for the end of therapy.

Box 4: Types of Individual Therapy

1. Cognitive Behavioral Therapy (CBT):

- Focuses on identifying and changing negative thought patterns and behaviors.
- Effective for anxiety, depression, and PTSD.

2. Psychodynamic Therapy:

- Explores unconscious processes and past experiences influencing current behavior.
- Useful for understanding emotional conflicts and relationship patterns.

3. Humanistic Therapy:

- Emphasizes personal growth and self-actualization.
- Techniques include person-centered therapy and Gestalt therapy.

4. Dialectical Behavior Therapy (DBT):

- A form of CBT designed for individuals with borderline personality disorder.
- Focuses on emotional regulation, interpersonal effectiveness, and distress tolerance.

5. Solution-Focused Brief Therapy (SFBT):

- Concentrates on finding solutions and setting achievable goals rather than exploring problems in-depth.
- Providing relapse prevention strategies.

Role of Nurses in Individual Psychotherapy

1. **Assessment and Evaluation:** Conduct initial assessments and use standardized tools to evaluate mental health.
2. **Building Therapeutic Relationships:** Establish trust, actively listen, and promote open communication.
3. **Psychoeducation:** Provide education on mental health, treatment options, and coping strategies.
4. **Implementation of Interventions:** Collaborate with therapists to implement treatment plans and support skill practice.
5. **Monitoring and Documentation:** Monitor progress, document changes, and communicate findings to the therapeutic team.
6. **Crisis Intervention:** Recognize signs of crisis, implement safety plans, and provide immediate support.
7. **Advocacy:** Advocate for patients' needs and encourage them to express treatment concerns.
8. **Family Involvement:** Engage family in therapy, offer support, and address dynamics affecting treatment.

9 Group Psychotherapy

Definition of Group Psychotherapy

Group psychotherapy involves a therapist working with a small group of individuals who share similar issues or concerns. This setting allows participants to learn from each other, provide support, and develop interpersonal skills (Box 5, Table 5). There are differences with individual therapies (Table 6), and different psychotherapeutic approaches fit better with different disorders (Table 7).

Table 5 Advantages and Disadvantages of Group Therapy

Advantages	Disadvantages
Sense of belonging—Reduces isolation.	Confidentiality concerns—Multiple members can affect privacy.
Multiple perspectives—Shared experiences.	Not suitable for severe conditions—May not be appropriate for individuals with serious psychiatric issues.
Encourages social skills—Develops interpersonal skills.	Group conflicts—Can hinder progress if issues arise within the group.
Cost-effective—More affordable than individual therapy.	Less individual attention—Limited focus on one-on-one needs.
Peer support—Fosters motivation and accountability.	Requires commitment—Needs consistent participation from members.

Table 6 Difference between individual therapy and group therapy

Aspect	Individual therapy	Group therapy
Focus	One-on-one sessions with the therapist	Multiple participants guided by a therapist
Customization	Tailored to the individual's unique needs	General interventions suited to the group's needs
Privacy	High confidentiality (client and therapist only)	Confidentiality can be more challenging due to group size
Attention	Focused, personalized attention from the therapist	Limited individual attention due to multiple participants
Pace	Progresses at the individual's pace	Progresses based on group dynamics and needs
Best for	Individuals with severe or complex issues, or those preferring privacy	People seeking peer support, shared experiences, and social skill development

Components of Group Therapy.

Group therapy involves multiple participants working together under the guidance of a therapist. It provides a supportive environment for shared experiences and healing.

A. **Group Formation.**

- Selection of participants based on shared concerns or disorders.
- Establishing group size and session structure.

B. **Group Rules and Guidelines.**

- Confidentiality agreement.
- Respectful communication and participation.

Table 7 Types of psychological interventions with indications

Type of Intervention	Indication
Cognitive behavioral therapy (CBT)	Depression, anxiety disorders
Dialectical behavior therapy (DBT)	Borderline personality disorder
Psychoanalysis	Unconscious conflicts in personality disorders
Psychodynamic therapy	Unresolved childhood trauma
Supportive therapy	Chronic mental illness (e.g., schizophrenia)
Group therapy	Social anxiety, substance use disorders
Family therapy	Family conflicts, parent–child relationship issues
Behavior therapy	Phobias, OCD
Mindfulness-based therapy	Stress, ASD, PTSD
Hypnotherapy	Pain management, PTSD
Electroconvulsive therapy (ECT)	Severe depression with suicidal risk
Play therapy	Childhood trauma, autism spectrum disorder
Art therapy	Expressing emotions in PTSD, trauma recovery

C. **Therapeutic Environment.**

- Creating a supportive, non-judgmental space.
- Encouraging open discussion and emotional expression.

D. **Group Dynamics and Interaction.**

- Members share experiences and provide support.
- Peer feedback and mutual problem-solving.

E. **Therapeutic Techniques.**

- Teaching coping skills and mental health knowledge through psychoeducation.
- Practicing role play technique for real-life interactions.
- Using Cognitive-Behavioral strategies to restructure thoughts and behaviors.

F. **Stages of Group Therapy.**

1. **Forming**—Establishing trust and setting goals.
2. **Storming**—Addressing disagreements and tensions.
3. **Norming**—Strengthening relationships and collaboration.
4. **Performing**—Active participation and progress.
5. **Adjourning**—Reflecting on progress and preparing for closure.

Techniques of Group Therapy

1. Psychoeducation: Educating group members on mental health topics and coping strategies.
2. Cognitive Restructuring: Challenging and modifying negative thought patterns.
3. Role-Playing: Practicing real-life situations to enhance coping and communication skills.
4. Guided Discussion: Facilitated conversations on emotions, experiences, and shared struggles.
5. Behavioral Rehearsal: Practicing new behaviors in a safe group setting.
6. Support and Feedback: Encouraging mutual support and constructive feedback among members.
7. Mindfulness and Relaxation: Teaching relaxation techniques to manage stress and anxiety.
8. Expressive Therapies: Using art, music, or movement to facilitate emotional expression.

Factors Contributing to the Group Therapy Process

1. Group Cohesion: Trust and belonging enhance effectiveness.
2. Interpersonal Learning: Learning from others' experiences and feedback.
3. Universality: Realizing you're not alone in struggles, reducing isolation.
4. Catharsis: Sharing emotions helps release suppressed feelings.
5. Imparting Information: Psychoeducation offers valuable knowledge and skills.
6. Altruism: Helping others fosters self-worth and growth.
7. Corrective Recapitulation of Family Dynamics: Reenacting past conflicts for emotional correction.
8. Development of Socializing Techniques: Practicing communication and interpersonal skills.
9. Existential Factors: Exploring personal meaning and life challenges.
10. Hope Instillation: Observing others' progress inspires optimism for change.

10 Role of Nurses in Group Psychotherapy

1. Facilitation and Support.

- Co-facilitate sessions and encourage participation.
- Create a welcoming, respectful environment for trust and communication.

2. Monitoring Group Dynamics.

- Observe and address conflicts or disruptive behaviors.
- Ensure members feel safe to share their experiences.

3. Psych Education and Skills Training.

- Provide education on mental health, coping strategies, and communication.
- Facilitate discussions to share insights and learn from one another.

4. **Encouraging Participation.**

- Motivate members to engage and support each other.
- Promote sharing personal experiences to foster connection.

5. **Documentation and Evaluation.**

- Document key themes, participation, and changes in attitudes or behaviors.
- Provide feedback to the lead therapist.

6. **Crisis Management.**

- Identify and manage crises during sessions.
- Implement interventions and ensure safety.

7. **Follow-Up Support.**

- Offer support to integrate therapy learnings into daily life.
- Encourage continued communication and connection outside sessions.

11 Psychiatric Nursing Interventions

Psychiatric nursing interventions are critical for supporting individuals with mental health conditions throughout their treatment process. These interventions are designed to promote recovery, improve coping skills, enhance emotional well-being, and facilitate communication. The key categories of psychiatric nursing interventions, along with specific examples and rationales for their use.

1. **Assessment Interventions**
   - Comprehensive Assessments: Gather mental health history and psychosocial factors.
     Rationale: Crucial for developing an effective treatment plan.

- Monitoring Vital Signs and Side Effects: Regular checks of physical health and medication effects.
  Rationale: Ensures safety and medication effectiveness.

2. **Therapeutic Communication**

- Active Listening: Reflective listening to understand patient concerns.
  Rationale: Builds a trusting therapeutic relationship.
- Empathy and Validation: Show understanding of patient emotions.
  Rationale: Encourages openness and rapport.

3. **Psychoeducation**

- Information on Mental Health: Educate on conditions, treatments, and coping strategies.
  Rationale: Empowers patients and families for informed decisions.
- Teaching Coping Skills: Instruct on relaxation, mindfulness, and problem-solving.
  Rationale: Encourages openness and rapport.

4. **Medication Management**

- Administering Medications: Ensure timely, accurate medication delivery.
  Rationale: Key to symptom control and treatment effectiveness.
- Medication Education: Provide info on dosage, side effects, and adherence.
  Rationale: Key to symptom control and treatment effectiveness.

5. **Crisis Intervention**

- Assessing for Risk: Evaluate for self-harm or harm to others.
  Rationale: Early intervention prevents crises.
- Safety Plans: Develop personalized plans for distress management.
  Rationale: Promotes self-efficacy in managing crises.

6. **Group Interventions**

- Facilitating Group Therapy: Co-facilitate sessions to promote peer support.
  Rationale: Fosters a sense of community and learning.
- Promoting Social Skills: Enhance interpersonal communication.
  Rationale: Improves relationships and support.

7. **Family Interventions**

- Involving Family Members: Educate and engage families in treatment.
  Rationale: Strengthens support systems and improves outcomes.
- Family Therapy: Facilitate communication and resolve family dynamics.
  Rationale: Reduces stressors impacting mental health..

8. **Behavioral Interventions**

    - Behavior Modification: Use reinforcement strategies to promote positive behaviors.
    - Rationale: Helps develop healthier habits and coping mechanisms.
    - Establishing Routine: Help create structured daily schedules.
      Rationale: Reduces anxiety and improves functioning.

9. **Cultural Competence**

    - Culturally Sensitive Care: Tailor interventions to cultural beliefs.
      Rationale: Enhances trust and engagement.
    - Understanding Cultural Norms: Explore cultural influences on mental health views.
      Rationale: Helps tailor interventions effectively.

10. **Discharge Planning**

    - Collaborating on Discharge Plans: Develop plans for post-hospital care and follow-up.
      Rationale: Ensures continuity of care and reduces relapse.
    - Connecting with Community Resources: Link patients to support groups and services.
      Rationale: Promotes long-term recovery.

Psychiatric Nursing Interventions in Psychotherapeutic Modalities

Psychiatric nurses play a critical role in implementing and supporting psychotherapeutic interventions. Their responsibilities vary depending on the type of therapy and the patient's needs. The key nursing interventions for different psychotherapeutic modalities:

1. Cognitive-Behavioral Therapy (CBT)

- Interventions:
- Assist in identifying negative thoughts.
- Encourage coping strategies and behavioral changes.
- Reinforce positive behaviors through goal setting.
- Teach relaxation techniques for anxiety.

Example: Help a depressed patient replace self-defeating thoughts with positive affirmations.

2. Psychoanalysis & Psychodynamic Therapy.

- Interventions:
- Build rapport to encourage self-exploration.
- Help recognize unconscious conflicts affecting behavior.
- Support emotional expression in a safe environment.
- Explore past relationships' impacts on current emotions.

Example: Encourage a patient to explore childhood experiences contributing to their fear of abandonment.

3. Humanistic Therapy (Client-Centered)

- Interventions:
- Provide unconditional positive regard for self-acceptance.
- Use active listening to validate emotions.
- Encourage self-exploration and personal growth.
- Assist in setting self-directed goals.

Example: Affirm strengths to a patient struggling with low self-esteem.

4. Group Therapy

- Interventions:
- Facilitate a supportive group environment.
- Encourage open communication and mutual support.
- Monitor group dynamics and individual participation.
- Guide conflict resolution.

Example: Lead a substance use support group for sharing coping strategies.

5. Family Therapy

- Interventions:
- Educate family on mental health conditions.
- Improve family communication patterns.
- Mediate conflicts and encourage problem-solving.
- Support boundary-setting and healthy interactions.

Example: Teach parents of an ADHD child to implement structured routines.

6. Dialectical Behavior Therapy (DBT).

- Interventions:
- Teach emotional regulation and distress tolerance.
- Support mindfulness and acceptance practices.

- Develop interpersonal effectiveness skills.
- Provide validation while encouraging change.

Example: Help a BPD patient use grounding techniques during emotional distress.

7. Behavioral Therapy (Exposure Therapy, Reinforcement).

- Interventions:
- Gradually expose patients to feared situations.
- Use positive reinforcement to encourage desired behaviors.
- Develop and implement behavior modification plans.

Example: Help a patient with phobia engage in graded exposure.

8. Psychopharmacological Therapy (Medication Management).

- Interventions:
- Educate on the purpose of psychotropic medication and its side effects.
- Monitor adherence and therapeutic effectiveness.
- Manage medication side effects.
- Advocate for patient safety in medication administration.

Example: Monitor antipsychotic medication side effects and report to psychiatrist.

9. Interpersonal Therapy (IPT).

- Interventions:
- Identify relationship patterns affecting mental health.
- Support conflict resolution skills.
- Encourage social support and connection-building.
- Guide role transition adjustments (e.g., grief, divorce).

Example: Help a patient rebuild relationships after social withdrawal.

Family Interventions/Therapy

Family interventions or family therapy is a therapeutic approach that involves working with couples and families to improve communication, resolve conflicts, and enhance overall functioning. These approaches utilize distinct theoretical frameworks and specialized techniques designed to address interpersonal dynamics and family systems, rather than simply extending individual therapy approaches to multiple people. Couple and family therapy is particularly useful when families face ongoing conflict, the mental illness of a member, or challenges related to divorce or blended family dynamics. By improving communication, fostering understanding, and strengthening relational bonds, these systemic approaches help couples and families develop healthier, more supportive, and resilient relationships (Box 6, 7).

Box 6: Key Concepts

- Family Systems Theory: This theory posits that a family functions as a complex system where each member influences and is influenced by the others. Changes in one part of the system can impact the whole family.
- Communication Patterns: Family therapy emphasizes the importance of effective communication among family members. Poor communication can lead to misunderstandings and conflicts.
- Roles and Dynamics: Families often have established roles and dynamics that can contribute to mental health issues. Identifying and modifying these roles can improve family functioning.
- Support and Strength: Family interventions leverage the support and strengths of family members to foster resilience and coping strategies.

Definition of Family Therapy: Family therapy is a form of psychological counseling that involves the entire family to improve communication, resolve conflicts, and strengthen relationships. It is based on the idea that family dynamics and interactions play a significant role in an individual's mental health and well-being.

12 Indications and Types of Family Therapy

The following list highlights key areas that may suggest the need for family therapy; however, these indicators are not exhaustive.

- **Mental Health Disorders**: Schizophrenia, bipolar disorder, depression, anxiety.
- **Behavioral Issues in Children & Adolescents**: Attention Deficit Hyperactivity Disorder (ADHD), Oppositional Defiant Disorder (ODD), and Conduct Disorders.
- **Marital & Relationship Conflicts**: Communication issues, divorce stress, domestic violence.
- **Parenting Challenges**: Single-parenting and raising children with special needs.
- **Chronic Illness/Disability**: Supporting ill family members and caregiving stress.
- **Trauma & Grief**: Coping with loss and grief.
- **Work & Financial Stress**: Job loss, workplace conflicts, and economic hardships.
- **Cultural & Generational Conflicts**: Parent-child value differences and acculturation struggles.
- **Blended Family Adjustments**: Step-parenting, co-parenting challenges, and sibling rivalry.
- **Addiction**: Alcohol/drug abuse, co-dependency.

13 Types of Family Therapy

Narrative Therapy

Narrative therapy is based on the premise that individuals construct stories about their lives, and these narratives shape their sense of identity and possibility. Central to narrative therapy is the practice of externalizing problems, viewing problems as separate from the person rather than as inherent personal defects. This linguistic shift allows clients to examine their relationship with problems from a new perspective. The therapeutic process focuses on re-authoring narratives, which means collaboratively exploring alternative stories that highlight client strengths, values, and preferred identities. Through techniques such as identifying unique outcomes, exploring absent but implicit values, and witnessing practices, clients develop more empowering life stories. Narrative therapy has been widely applied across individual, family, and community settings, particularly in contexts where cultural and social factors significantly influence identity and well-being.

Family Systems Therapy

Family systems therapy emerged from the work of theorists including Murray Bowen, Salvador Minuchin, Virginia Satir, and Jay Haley during the mid-twentieth century. This approach conceptualizes individuals within the context of relational and systemic patterns rather than as isolated units. Psychological problems are understood not as residing within a single person but as emerging from interaction patterns, family structures, communication styles, and relational dynamics within the family system. Different schools within family systems therapy have developed distinct emphases, such as *structural family therapy* (Minuchin) focuses on hierarchies and boundaries; *strategic family therapy* (Haley) emphasizes problem-solving interventions; and systemic family therapy (Bowen) addresses multigenerational patterns and differentiation of self. Modern family therapists emphasize working collaboratively with families, recognizing that each family member may have a valid but different perspective on their situation. Rather than claiming to know the "right" answer, therapists help families create new understandings and interaction patterns together. In this updated view, the therapist is seen as part of the therapeutic process, someone who participates with the family rather than as an external expert who observes and directs from outside the family system.

Solution Focused Brief Therapy (SFBT)

Solution Focused Brief Therapy (SFBT) emphasizes clients' existing strengths and resources rather than focusing on problems, deficits, or pathology. SFBT treatment is brief, structured, and goal-oriented. It identifies exceptions, such as times when the problem is absent or less severe, and builds practical solutions from these successes. Core techniques of SFBT include the *miracle question* (asking clients to imagine life after the problem is solved), *scaling questions* (rating progress and goals numerically), and *exception-finding* (exploring when and how the problem does not occur). These techniques help clients envision possibilities and implement concrete steps toward change. The therapist adopts a collaborative, facilitative stance, trusting in the client's capacity to identify workable solutions.

Goals of Family Therapy

1. Improve Communication—Help family members express their thoughts and feelings openly and effectively.
2. Enhance Problem-Solving Skills—Equip families with strategies to manage conflicts and stress.
3. Strengthen Relationships—Foster emotional bonds and trust among family members.
4. Promote Understanding and Empathy—Encourage family members to understand each other's perspectives.
5. Address Dysfunctional Patterns—Identify and modify negative behaviors affecting family dynamics.
6. Support Individual and Collective Growth—Encourage personal development while maintaining family harmony.
7. Prevent and Manage Crises—Equip families with coping mechanisms for challenges such as divorce, illness, or loss.

Box 7: Principles of Family Therapy

- Systems Perspective—The family is viewed as an interconnected system where changes in one member affect the whole.
- Holistic Approach—Addresses emotional, behavioral, and relational aspects of the family unit.
- Collaboration—The therapist works with the entire family rather than focusing on one individual.
- Active Participation—Family members are encouraged to engage in discussions and therapeutic exercises.
- Flexibility and Adaptability—Therapy is tailored to each family's unique needs and dynamics.

Techniques of Family Therapy

1. Structural Family Therapy (SFT) focuses on reorganizing family structure and hierarchies.
2. Strategic Family Therapy uses directive techniques to alter specific problematic interactions.
3. Bowenian Family Therapy emphasizes emotional differentiation and reducing anxiety within family relationships.
4. Cognitive-Behavioral Family Therapy (CBFT) uses cognitive and behavioral techniques to change dysfunctional thought patterns and behaviors.
5. Narrative Therapy encourages family members to reframe their personal and collective stories to promote healing.
6. Genogram Analysis uses family tree diagrams to analyze generational patterns and emotional connections.
7. Communication Training enhances open and effective communication within the family.
8. Role-Playing and rehearsal help family members practice new ways of interacting.

Role of Family Interventions in Mental Health Care

- Family therapy considers the individual within the context of their family, recognizing the interdependence of relationships and mental health.
- By involving family members, individuals may feel more supported and understood, leading to better treatment adherence and outcomes.
- Many mental health issues have roots in family dynamics, and addressing these can lead to improved functioning and symptom reduction.
- Family therapy can be an effective intervention during crises, helping families navigate acute stress and support one another.
- Families that participate in therapy often develop lasting skills and healthier communication patterns, which can prevent future conflicts and promote resilience.

Role of Nurses in Family Interventions or Family Therapy.

The role of nurses in family interventions and therapy is critical to promoting mental health and facilitating effective family dynamics. Nurses bring unique skills and perspectives to family therapy, enhancing the therapeutic process and supporting families in their journey toward improved mental health. The key aspects of a nurse's role in family interventions:

1. **Assessment**
   - Evaluate family dynamics, communication patterns, and challenges.
   - Identify strengths and mental health concerns.
2. **Education**
   - Provide information on mental health conditions & treatments.
   - Teach coping strategies & effective communication.
3. **Support & Advocacy**
   - Offer emotional support & advocate for family needs.
   - Connect families to additional community resources.
4. **Facilitating Therapy Sessions**
   - Assist as co-therapists in sessions.
   - Create a safe space for open discussions.
5. **Monitoring Progress**
   - Track improvements in relationships & mental health.
   - Adjust interventions as needed.
6. **Crisis Intervention**
   - Handle conflicts & mental health crises.
   - Develop safety plans for at-risk family members.
7. **Promoting Family Involvement**
   - Encourage participation in treatment planning.
   - Strengthen family support systems.
8. **Reflective Practice**
   - Engage in self-reflection to enhance care.
   - Continue education in family therapy & mental health nursing.

Psychiatric nurses support these psychotherapeutic modalities by providing tailored interventions, enhancing coping mechanisms, and fostering a holistic approach to mental health treatment.

Sample Short Answer Questions

1. Write down the classifications of Psychotropic Medications.
2. Write down the types of antipsychotics, antidepressants, mood stabilizers, Anxiolytics and Sedative-Hypnotics.
3. Write down the indications of antipsychotics, antidepressants, mood stabilizers, Anxiolytics and Sedative-Hypnotics.

4. Write down the side effects of antipsychotics, antidepressants, mood stabilizers, Anxiolytics and Sedative-Hypnotics.
5. What is ECT with its indications and contraindications?
6. What is family therapy?
7. Write down the indications and types of family therapy.
8. What is psychotherapy with its goal?
9. Write down the classification and indications of psychotherapy.
10. What is individual/group therapy?
11. Write down the factors contributing group therapy process.

Sample Essay Questions

1. Describe the extrapyramidal symptoms of antipsychotics.
2. How will you prepare an ECT patient?
3. Explain the complications of ECT
4. Explain the goals and principles of family therapy.
5. Explain the techniques of family therapy.
6. Explain the stages of group therapy.
7. Describe the advantages & disadvantages of group therapy.
8. Explain the role of nurses of individual/group therapy.
9. Explain the techniques of group therapy.
10. Explain the Psychiatric Nursing Interventions.

Sample Multiple Choice Questions (MCQ) *and* Sample Best Answer Questions

Psychiatric nursing interventions include-			What is the primary purpose of psychopharmacology in psychiatric care?		
T	a)	Includes therapeutic communication.		a)	To cure mental health disorders
F	b)	Only involves medication.	✓	b)	To manage symptoms of mental health disorders
T	c)	Crisis intervention is included.		c)	To provide psychotherapy
F	d)	Education is unnecessary.		d)	To replace other therapeutic interventions
T	e)	Supports recovery and coping.			

Suggetsed Reading

American Psychiatric Association. (2022). *Diagnostic and statistical manual of mental disorders* (5th ed., text rev ed., p. DSM-5-TR). American Psychiatric Publishing.
Beck, J. S., Beck, A. T., & Beck, J. S. (2011). *Cognitive behavior therapy: Basics and beyond* (ed. ed.).
Corey, G. (2013). *Theory and practice of counseling and psychotherapy*. Brooks/Cole Cengage Learning.
Davison, G. C., Neale, J. M., & Hindman, D. (1996). *Abnormal psychology* (p. 710). Wiley.
Fehr, S. S. (2014). *Introduction to group therapy: A practical guide*. Routledge.
Gelder, M. G., Lopez-Ibor, J. J., & Andreasen, N. C. (2003). New Oxford textbook of psychiatry, *Volume 2*. Oxford University Press.
Minuchin, S., & Fishman, H. C. (1981). *Family therapy techniques*. Harvard University Press.
Prochaska, J. O., & Norcross, J. C. (2018). *Systems of psychotherapy: A transtheoretical analysis*. Oxford University Press.
Shaffer, J. B., & Galinsky, M. D. (1989). Models of group therapy. Prentice-Hall, Inc.
Wood, J. C., & Wood, M. (2008). *Therapy 101: A brief look at modern psychotherapy techniques and how they can help*. New Harbinger Publications.

Chapter 4
Therapeutic Communication and Therapeutic Relationship

Kulsuma Akter and S. M. Yasir Arafat

Abstract In psychiatric nursing, therapeutic communication is a cornerstone of effective nursing practice, building a foundation of trust and collaboration between patient and nurse, especially in psychiatric wards where patients exhibit aggressive and non-cooperative behavior. It begins with the idea of the therapeutic use of self as a tool for diagnosing mental disorders. This chapter focuses on how empathetic behavior from nurses help patients in improving relaxation, motivation, and their clinical outcomes. This chapter highlights key techniques of therapeutic communication that would make interaction more effective and meaningful, while also addressing barriers and strategies to overcome them. By combining these ideas, this chapter provides clear guidance for nurses to foster caring, supportive relationships that improve patient well-being and promote positive outcomes in psychiatric nursing practice.

Keywords Therapeutic use of self · Empathy · Nurse-patient relationship · Therapeutic communication

1 Therapeutic Use of Self

Therapeutic use of self refers to how nurses interconnect their own self-concept with their patients through speaking, listening, and building rapport as a part of the therapeutic process. It involves the ability to connect authentically with patients while maintaining professional boundaries and focusing on their needs. It is an essential therapeutic tool in establishing an effective nurse-patient relationship. It helps to

K. Akter
Department of Nursing and Health Science, Jashore University of Science and Technology, Jashore, Bangladesh

S. M. Y. Arafat (✉)
Department of Psychiatry, Bangladesh Specialized Hospital, Dhaka, Bangladesh
e-mail: arafatdmc62@gmail.com

S. M. Y. Arafat and H. Akter (eds.), *Psychiatric Nursing in Bangladesh*, Mental Health Systems and Policy in Low- and Middle-Income Countries,
https://doi.org/10.1007/978-981-95-8501-4_4

improve nurses' practice skills to perceive their patients with different clinical situations. Furthermore, it engages nurses in understanding patients' insights, perceptions, values, and attitudes. While patients identify nurses as more approachable and professional, Patients feel empowered to explore their feelings, experiences, and understanding related to their disorder. Thus, it makes nurses more conscious of their roles and the application of an empathetic approach in patient care, which leads to quality nursing care and positive clinical outcomes.

2 Key Components of Therapeutic Use of Self

1. Self-Awareness

Nurses recognize and are aware of their emotions, values, strengths, and limitations to interact effectively with patients. For example, understanding that the pattern of speech delivery may discomfort patients, and adjustment may be necessary.

2. Authenticity

Being genuine and transparent in interactions with patients fosters trust and openness. Sharing appropriate personal experiences that relate to a patient's struggles to create a sense of connection.

3. Empathy

Understanding patients' feelings and experiences from their perspective for establishing a strong therapeutic alliance. For example, understanding cancer patients' concerns about chemotherapy-related hair loss and discussing supportive coping strategies.

4. Boundaries

The interaction must be maintained by a professional nurse–patient relationship. For example, setting limits on self-disclosure to keep the focus on the patient.

5. Active Listening

Fully focusing on the patient's words, tone, and nonverbal cues without judgment. For example, maintaining eye contact, nodding, and summarizing to demonstrate attentive understanding.

6. Flexibility

Applying care strategies to meet patients' unique needs. For example, modifying communication styles to increase patient self-awareness.

Empathy

Empathy encompasses the ability to understand situations from the patients' point of view, interpret their emotional state, and foster effective interpersonal interactions. It is such an attribute that can motivate nurses care giving behavior. Empathy begins in early childhood and gradually matures over time. Evidence shows that disorders resulting from empathy deficiency, including antisocial, borderline, and narcissistic personality disorders; autism spectrum disorders; and schizophrenia can be identified in early childhood. In the mental healthcare context, the establishment of an effective nurse–patient relationship between nurse and patient largely depends on the application of empathy. Indeed, empathetic ability helps nurses to own a nonjudgmental approach and facilitate it from the orientation phases to all subsequent phases of the therapeutic relationship and positive impact on job satisfaction and patient outcomes. Therefore, during the orientation phase of the therapeutic relationship, nurses show their interest in understanding the actual situation.

Importance of Empathy in Psychiatric Nursing

1. **Building Trust**. Empathy helps in establishing trust between the nurse and the patient.
2. **Developing therapeutic relationships.** Empathy is considered an important aspect to establish the patient–nurse relationship. With empathy, nurses can show their confident attitudes toward patients with mental illness.
3. **Improving patients' positive clinical outcomes**. Research has shown that a higher level of empathetic concern among nurses is associated with positive clinical outcomes and reduced medication errors. Furthermore, it enhances the patient's relaxation, motivation, and cooperative behavior.
4. **Supporting Coping Strategies**: Patients who are exposed to higher empathic support tend to lower anxiety, enhanced self-perception, and diminished depression and hostility.
5. **Facilitating emotional expression**: Empathy encourages patients to express their emotions and concerns, which can be crucial for their healing process.
6. **Fostering nurses' competency and professional satisfaction.** Being empathetic, nurses can enhance the effectiveness of any nursing interventions with less psychological stress and professional burnout. Advanced education in psychiatric nursing, more experience, and a higher level of attitude were identified as significant predictors that enhanced nurses' empathetic ability toward patients with mental disorders.

3 Nurse–Patient Relationship

The nurse–patient relationship is a therapeutic and professional interaction between a nurse and a patient, aimed at promoting the patient's well-being, recovery, and overall mental and physical health. It is based on genuineness, trust, respect, empathy, confidentiality, and professional boundaries to ensure that the patient feels safe and supported while receiving care (Fig. 1).

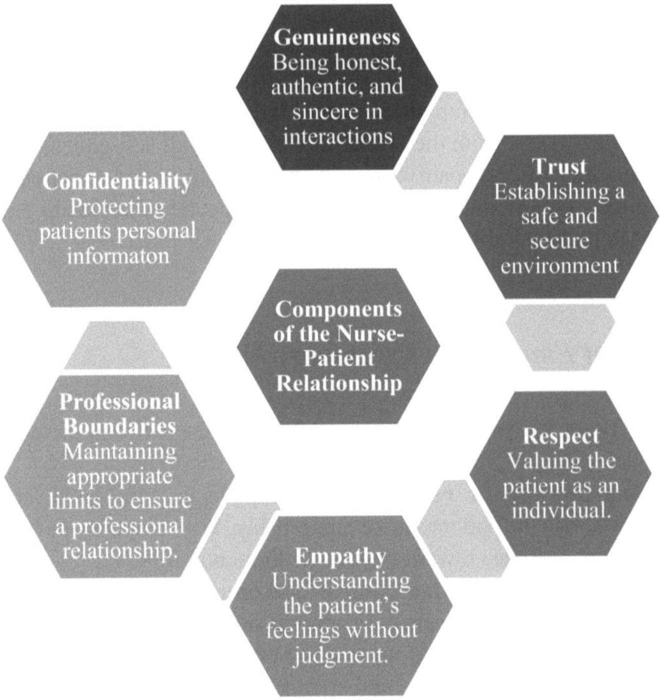

Fig. 1 Components of the nurse–client relationship

Nurses Roles in Therapeutic Relationship

Nurse–patient relationship is a significant component in establishing therapeutic communication, especially in a psychiatric patient care unit. Characteristics of nurse–patient relationship are presented in Box 1.

Hildegard Peplau (Interpersonal Relations in Nursing) identifies six subroles of nurses establishing nurse–patient relationship are as follows:

Stranger Both nurse and patient are strangers to each other. Nurse accepts each patient as they are.

Nurse teacher who educate patient about medication and inhaler techniques to improve health conditions.

Clinical nurse usually assesses patients' condition, administers medication, and performs invasive procedures.

Nurse manager is responsible for maintaining a patient care environment with adequate medicines and equipment in a patient care unit where the patient can feel secure and safe.

Social agent role of nurses promotes social interaction with different groups by using social skills.

Counselor nurse helps patients in decision-making, strategies in minimizing stress, and how to resolve a crisis.

Box 1. Characteristics of Nurse–patient Relationship

1. Consistency and Reliability: Maintaining a consistent approach in interactions helps in building trust and predictability in the relationship.
2. Boundaries: Maintaining professional boundaries.
3. Mutual Respect: Valuing the patient's thoughts, feelings, and experiences, fostering an environment of respect.
4. Empathy: Empathetic nurses can understand patient's emotional state and create a comfortable environment
5. Confidentiality: Ensuring the patients' information remains secured.
6. Focus on the Patient's Needs: Prioritizing the patient's needs and problem-solving strategies.

Phases of the Nurse–Patient Relationship

The nurse–patient relationship is a key component of psychiatric care, fostering trust and collaboration to support the patient's recovery. Tasks of nurse patient relationship have been categorized into four phases: pre-interaction, orientation, working, and termination. Each phase has unique characteristics and goals compared with others. Table 1 includes the major nursing tasks during each phase of nurse–patient relationship.

Pre-Interaction Phase

This phase begins before the nurse's first contact with the patient. The nurse prepares emotionally and gathers relevant patient information. For example: A nurse reviews the chart of a patient diagnosed with bipolar disorder and plans how to approach the initial interaction.

Key Features

- Reviewing the patient's medical and psychological history.
- Reflecting on personal attitudes or feelings that may influence the relationship.
- Identifying potential challenges and planning strategies for care.

  Preparing oneself for working.

Table 1 Phases of nurse–patient relationship

Phase	Tasks
1. Pre-Interaction Phase	• Preparing for the interaction by gathering information and reflecting on one's own feelings • Example: Reviewing the patient's medical history
2. Orientation Phase	• Introducing oneself • Building trust and rapport • Establishing confidentiality and ensuring patient safety • Identifying the patient's current needs, strength and weakness • Developing a nursing care plan • Example: Greeting the patient and creating a comfortable environment for the patient
3. Working Phase	• Exploring problems and encouraging the patient to express feelings • Implementing plan into action and evaluate the outcomes of nursing action • Teaching coping strategies and working towards goals • Example: Discussing stress management techniques with an anxious patient
4. Termination Phase	• Concluding the relationship by summarizing progress and discussing future steps • Helping the patient prepare for independence • Example: "You've made great progress. Let's review the skills you can use moving forward."

Orientation Phase

It begins during the first contact with the patient. In this phase, the nurse and the patient get introduction about each other. During the orientation phase, nurses' main concern is to identify patients' problems and motivations for care and treatment. It is very important for nurses to realize each patient beyond individual social, cultural, and anxiety levels.

Key Features

- Introducing yourself and explaining your role.
- Creating a favorable environment.
- Building trust through active listening, empathy, and nonjudgmental behavior.
- Setting goals and outlining the structure of the relationship.
- Building rapport for nursing intervention.
- Discussing confidentiality and its boundaries.

Working Phase

Utmost therapeutic work is applied throughout the working phase. The nurse and patient work collaboratively to explore problems and their thoughts by aligning perception, feeling, and action.

Key Features

- Encouraging the patient to express feelings and concerns.
- Assisting the patient in identifying problems and formulating solutions.
- Providing emotional support and implementing interventions.
- Facilitating patient learning and behavioral changes.

Termination Phase

It is one of the most important phases of therapeutic relationship where nurses are determined for patient termination by evaluating the progress status and attainment of a specific goal. In this phase, the patient is either discharged from the hospital, discharges oneself, or even dies.

Key Features

- Reviewing progress made during the relationship.
- Reinforcing coping strategies and skills learned.
- Providing resources for continued support if needed.
- Saying goodbye and addressing feelings of separation.

Following these phases ensures a structured and therapeutic approach to patient care. It helps build trust, set clear expectations, and support the patient's journey toward recovery. It prepares the patient for independence and self-care in managing their mental health. By progressing through these phases, nurses create a safe, supportive, and effective environment for therapeutic relationships.

4 Therapeutic Communications

Therapeutic communication is a process by which face-to-face interaction and purposeful exchange of information take place between the nurse and the patient that focuses on advancing the patient's physical and mental well-being. In a psychiatric nursing care setting, nurses consciously use specific strategies to interact with the patient and encourage the patient to express their feelings through verbal or nonverbal communication. The importance of therapeutic communication is discussed in Box 2. Nurses engage with patients to identify problems and provide holistic care, support, and recovery.

Box 2. Importance of Therapeutic Communication

- Builds Trust: Effective communication fosters a safe environment where patients feel comfortable sharing their thoughts and emotions.
- Facilitates Understanding: Effective communication helps patients understand their conditions, treatment options, and adapting coping strategies.

- Enhances Engagement: Patients who feel heard and understood are more likely to engage in their treatment plans and take an active role in their recovery.
- Promotes Emotional Expression: Encouraging patients to express their feelings can lead to emotional relief and insight into their experiences.

For building effective communication with patients, nurses need to focus on the different therapeutic techniques included in Box 3.

Box 3. Techniques of Therapeutic Communication

1. **Active Listening**:
   - Fully focus on the patient, demonstrating attentiveness through verbal and non-verbal cues.
   - *Example*: Nodding, maintaining eye contact, and reflecting on what the patient says.
2. **Empathy**:
   - Show understanding and compassion for the patient's feelings and experiences.
   - *Example*: "It sounds like you're feeling overwhelmed; that must be really difficult for you."
3. **Open-Ended Questions**:
   - Encourage patients for sharing their experience by asking questions that cannot be answered with a simple "yes" or "no."
   - *Example*: "can you explain the location and radiation of your pain?
4. **Clarification**:
   - Help patients clarify the feelings when they express thoughts and doubts.
   - *Example*: "Could you explain how much water you drink within 24 h?
5. **Reflection**:
   - Mirror back the patient's feelings or statements to show understanding and encourage further exploration.
   - *Example*: "It sounds like you're saying that you feel anxious about the future."
6. **Summarization**:
   - Summarize key points from the conversation to support your understanding and ensure its' accuracy.
   - *Example*: "To summarize, you've been feeling anxious about earthquake, and it's affecting your sleep."
7. **Non-Verbal Communication**:
   - Be aware about of body language, facial expressions, as they can significantly impact communication.

- *Example*: Observe physical appearance, body movement and posture, and voice.

5 Barriers to Therapeutic Communication

Therapeutic communication in psychiatric nursing requires careful attention to avoid barriers that may hinder its effectiveness. These barriers can arise from the patient, nurse, or environment. Different communication barriers and strategies to overcome these barriers are presented in Table 2.

Take Home Message

- Understanding patient feeling and experience from their perspective is empathy
- Nurse-patient relationship is guided by professional characteristics and phases
- Therapeutic communication has sets of skills and phases
- Nurses should be aware of the barriers of therapeutic communications and their potential strategies to overcome

Sample Short Answer Questions

1. What is the therapeutic use of self, with its importance?
2. Write down the key components of the therapeutic use of self.
3. Write down the significance of empathy in nursing.
4. Write down the characteristics of a Therapeutic Relationship.
5. Write down the key components of the Nurse–Client Relationship.

Sample Essay Questions

1. Explain the Phases of the Nurse–Patient Relationship
2. Describe the role of nurses in establishing and maintaining the therapeutic relationship.
3. Explain the techniques of therapeutic communication
4. Explain the phases of therapeutic communication
5. Explain the barriers to therapeutic communication and strategies to overcome these barriers

Sample Multiple Choice Questions (MCQ) and Sample Best Answer

Table 2 Barriers to therapeutic communication

Categories of communication barrier	Description of barriers	Strategies to overcome barriers
1.1. Patient-Related Barriers	Language barriers Language jargons Faulty language translations Individual differences in expression and perception Anxiety, anger, or fear of initiating speaking Conditions like schizophrenia, dementia, or delirium can impair thought processes and communication Various cultural customs and beliefs	Avoid jargon during communication Language must be simple and clear Respect and acknowledge cultural differences
1.2. Nurse-Related Barriers	Lack of self-awareness Lack of attention Poor listening skills Displaying bias Inadequate training Information overload Discomfort due to illness	Draw complete attention Show genuine interest through verbal and nonverbal cues Limitations of hearing must be kept in mind Information overload must be kept in mind
1.3. Environmental Barriers	Poor lighting Loud noise Lack of privacy Unfamiliar and uncomfortable setting Unhygienic surroundings Inappropriate distance	Good lighting Noise must be kept at the lowest possible level Comfortable sitting arrangement Hygienic and odor-free environment
1.4. Interaction-Related Barriers	Conflicting massage Use of Medical Jargon Neglecting nonverbal cues like body language or facial expressions Stereotyping approach Limited time Inappropriate channels Lack of poor feedback	Avoid complex terms and medical jargons while communicating with the patient Use appropriate channel of communication Allocate sufficient time for meaningful interactions Give effective feedback

Therapeutic Use of Self involves-			Which of the following is a barrier to therapeutic communication?		
T	(a)	Requires self-awareness and intentionality		(a)	Showing empathy
F	(b)	Focuses on meeting nurses' emotional needs	✓	(b)	Using medical jargon

(continued)

(continued)

Therapeutic Use of Self involves-			Which of the following is a barrier to therapeutic communication?		
T	(c)	Building trust is fundamental		(c)	Active listening
F	(d)	Sharing personal problems is key		(d)	Quiet environment
T	(e)	Clear boundaries are essential			

Suggested Reading

Alkan, A. (2017). The effects of Nurses' empathy skills on attitudes towards patients with cancer. *Journal of Clinical and Experimental Investigations., 8*(2), 61–65. https://doi.org/10.5799/jcei.333383

Derksen, F., Olde Hartman, T. C., Van Dijk, A., Plouvier, A., Bensing, J., & Lagro-Janssen, A. (2017). Consequences of the presence and absence of empathy during consultations in primary care: A focus group study with patients. *Patient Education and Counseling., 100*(5), 987–993. https://doi.org/10.1016/j.pec.2016.12.003

Duarte, J., & Pinto-Gouveia, J. (2017). Empathy and feelings of guilt experienced by nurses: A cross-sectional study of their role in burnout and compassion fatigue symptoms. *Applied Nursing Research., 35*, 42–47. https://doi.org/10.1016/j.apnr.2017.02.006

Håkansson Eklund, J., Holmström, I. K., Ollén Lindqvist, A., Sundler, A. J., Hochwälder, J., & Marmstål, H. L. (2019). Empathy levels among nursing students: A comparative cross-sectional study. *Nursing Open., 6*(3), 983–989. https://doi.org/10.1002/nop2.280

Hamed, W. E., Babegi, A. S., Elamin, H. A. M., Kamel, N. A., Escolano-Castillo, A. M., Dailah, H. G., et al. (2025). Stigmatizing attitudes and predictors of empathy toward mentally ill patients among psychiatric and mental health nurses. *BMC Nursing, 24*(1), 454. https://doi.org/10.1186/s12912-025-02926-z

Richmond, J. S., Dragatsi, D., Stiebel, V., Rozel, J. S., & Rasimas, J. J. (2021). American Association for emergency psychiatry recommendations to address psychiatric staff shortages in emergency settings. *PS, 72*(4), 437–443. https://doi.org/10.1176/appi.ps.201900501

Yuguero, O., Ramon Marsal, J., Esquerda, M., Vivanco, L., & Soler-González, J. (2017). Association between low empathy and high burnout among primary care physicians and nurses in Lleida. *Spain. European Journal of General Practice., 23*(1), 4–10. https://doi.org/10.1080/13814788.2016.1233173

Yuguero, O., Forné, C., Esquerda, M., Pifarré, J., Abadías, M. J., & Viñas, J. (2017). Empathy and burnout of emergency professionals of a health region: A cross-sectional study. *Medicine, 96*(37), e8030. https://doi.org/10.1097/MD.0000000000008030

Walocha, E., Tomaszewski, K. A., Wilczek-Ruzyczka, E., & Walocha, J. (2013). Empathy and burnout among physicians of different specialities. *Folia Medica Cracoviensia, 53*(2), 35–42.

Chapter 5
Care of Clients with Schizophrenia and Other Psychotic Disorders

Atiqul Haq Mazumder and S. M. Yasir Arafat

Abstract Schizophrenia and other psychotic disorders represent some of the most complex and severe mental health conditions, characterized by a profound disruption in an individual's thoughts, perceptions, emotions, and behavior. This chapter provides a comprehensive and practical guide for psychiatric nurses on the evidence-based care of clients experiencing psychosis. It begins by defining key terms and outlining the diagnostic criteria for schizophrenia and related disorders. It explores the multifactorial etiology of psychosis, integrating the evidence on genetic, neurobiological, and environmental risk factors. A significant focus is placed on the nursing process, detailing holistic assessment strategies and tailored interventions for managing positive, negative, and cognitive symptoms. The critical role of the nurse in safely administering and monitoring antipsychotics, including the management of common side effects, is examined. Furthermore, the chapter emphasizes the importance of psychosocial interventions, patient and family education, and relapse prevention strategies to support long-term recovery and successful community reintegration. Through clinical vignettes, flowcharts, and practical tables, this chapter equips nurses with the essential knowledge and skills to deliver compassionate, competent, and effective care to this vulnerable population.

Keywords Schizophrenia · Psychotic disorders · Nursing care · Antipsychotic agents · Mental health recovery · Psychiatric nursing · Delusions · Hallucinations · Relapse prevention · Community mental health

A. H. Mazumder
Department of Psychiatry, Faculty of Medicine, Research Unit of Clinical Medicine, University of Oulu, Oulu, Finland

S. M. Y. Arafat (✉)
Department of Psychiatry, Bangladesh Specialized Hospital, Dhaka, Bangladesh
e-mail: arafatdmc62@gmail.com

S. M. Y. Arafat and H. Akter (eds.), *Psychiatric Nursing in Bangladesh*, Mental Health Systems and Policy in Low- and Middle-Income Countries,
https://doi.org/10.1007/978-981-95-8501-4_5

1 Introduction

Psychotic disorders are a group of serious illnesses that affect the mind. They make it difficult for someone to think clearly, make good judgments, respond emotionally, communicate effectively, understand reality, and behave appropriately. When symptoms are severe, people with psychotic disorders have trouble staying in touch with reality and are often unable to meet the ordinary demands of daily life. Schizophrenia is the most common and well-known of these disorders, but the spectrum also includes schizoaffective disorder, delusional disorder, brief psychotic disorder, and others. Nursing management requires a sophisticated understanding of not only the shared features of psychosis but also the unique presentation and course of each specific disorder.

Case Vignette-1

Mr. K, a 22-year-old university student, is brought to the psychiatric unit by his concerned family. Over the past eight months, his academic performance has deteriorated, and he has withdrawn from friends and hobbies. For the last two months, his behavior has become increasingly unusual; he isolates himself in his room, is often heard muttering, and expresses a firm belief that his professors are "spies" sent to steal his groundbreaking ideas. He also reports hearing a voice comment on his actions and warns him not to trust his family. On assessment, Mr. K appears disheveled, suspicious, and exhibits a flat affect and disorganized speech. He has poor nutrition and has lost significant weight. This combination of positive symptoms (delusions, hallucinations), negative symptoms (flat affect, avolition), and severe functional impairment is characteristic of schizophrenia.

Case Vignette-2

Mrs. Z is a 42-year-old married Bangladeshi woman from a middle-class Dhaka household, working as a bank officer and mother to two children. Her family attributed her initial withdrawal and insomnia to stress or jinn (spirit possession), consulting a local healer. Her presentation worsened with overt psychotic manifestations: she became convinced male colleagues were conspiring to ruin her reputation using black magic (kala jadu), believing she heard them plotting during calls. She covered mirrors at home, fearing the evil eye (nazar), and grew suspicious of her husband, accusing him of collusion. This caused severe marital strain and neglect of her children, compelling her husband to seek help from a private clinic in the city.

Her case highlights barriers like stigma, supernatural attributions of mental illness, and delayed psychiatric care. Treatment must be culturally nuanced, integrating antipsychotics with family psychoeducation, addressing cultural beliefs. The central challenge is maintaining her crucial employment and family roles amidst significant social pressure, requiring a support system to ensure adherence and prevent relapse in a resource-constrained environment.

Concept

The term schizophrenia, from the Greek roots schizo (split) and phren (mind), was coined by Eugen Bleuler in 1908. He used it to describe the "splitting" or fragmentation of psychic functions. While much of the historical understanding of psychosis is rooted in the study of schizophrenia, it has provided the foundational concepts for understanding the entire spectrum of psychotic disorders. Figure 1 provides a historical perspective of schizophrenia.

Nosology

Psychotic disorders are grouped in both the *Diagnostic and Statistical Manual of Mental Disorders* (DSM-5) and the *International Classification of Diseases* (ICD-11). The key distinctions among them often relate to symptom duration, the types of symptoms present, and whether a mood disorder is also present (Table 1).

2 Understanding Psychotic Disorders

Psychosis

Psychosis is not a diagnosis in itself but a syndrome composed of several key symptoms. The hallmark features are delusions and hallucinations. A delusion is a false, unshakable belief that is firmly held despite clear evidence or reasoning to the contrary, not shared by community members, and not explained by educational, cultural, or religious background. A hallucination is a sensory perception in the absence of an external stimulus. It is a percept to the corresponding sensory organ without any external stimuli. It can affect any of the five senses and is experienced as real by the individual. Understanding these core symptoms is fundamental to recognizing psychosis (See Boxes 1, 2).

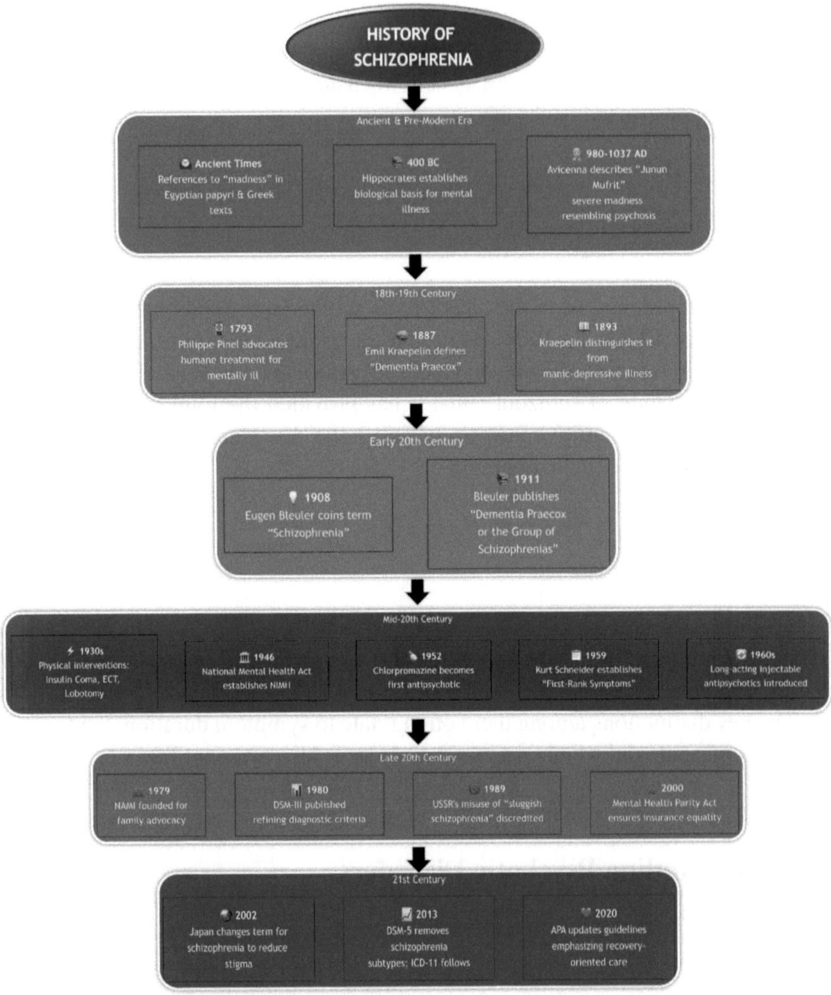

Fig. 1 Historical perspective of schizophrenia

Table 1 Comparison of nosology of primary psychotic disorders

S. no	DSM-5 (Schizophrenia spectrum and other psychotic disorders)	ICD-11 (Schizophrenia or other primary psychotic disorders)
1	Schizophrenia	Schizophrenia
2	Schizophreniform disorder	Acute and transient psychotic disorder
3	Schizoaffective disorder	Schizoaffective disorder
4	Delusional disorder	Delusional disorder
5	Brief psychotic disorder	Acute and transient psychotic disorder
6	Schizotypal (personality) disorder	Schizotypal disorder

Box 1 Common Delusions

- **Persecutory:** Belief that one is being plotted against, spied on, or harmed.
  - Example: "My coworkers are poisoning my food to get my job."
- **Grandiose:** Belief in one's exaggerated importance, power, or identity.
  - Example: "I am a messenger from God with a special mission."
- **Referential:** Belief that neutral environmental cues are personally directed at oneself.
  - Example: "The news anchor on TV is sending me secret messages."
- **Somatic:** Beliefs involving bodily functions or sensations.
  - Example: "My internal organs have turned to stone."
- **Erotomanic:** The belief that another person, often of higher status, is in love with them.
  - Example: "A famous actor is secretly in love with me."
- **Nihilistic (Cotard's Delusion):** The belief that oneself, a part of one's body, or the world does not exist or has been destroyed.
  - Example: "I am already dead and this is just a dream."
- **Delusions of Control:** The belief that one's thoughts, feelings, or actions are being controlled by an external force.
  - Example: "An alien is controlling my arm and making me write this."
- **Jealous (Othello Syndrome):** The unfounded belief that one's spouse or partner is unfaithful, often based on trivial or misinterpreted evidence.
  - Example: "I know my husband is cheating because he came home two minutes late."
- **Delusions of Guilt or Sin:** An unfounded belief that one is responsible for a terrible crime or disaster.
  - Example: "The earthquake on the other side of the world happened because I had a bad thought.

Box 2 Common Hallucinations

- **Auditory:** Hearing voices or other sounds that are not present. This is the most common type in schizophrenia.
  - Example: "I hear someone always talking about me when no one is around."

- **Visual:** Seeing people, objects, or patterns that are not there.
  - Example: "I sometimes see a supernatural being floating inside my room."
- **Tactile:** Feeling sensations on the skin, such as insects crawling (formication) or being touched.
  - Example: "I often sense some maggots crawling beneath my skin."
- **Olfactory:** Smelling odors that no one else detects, often unpleasant ones like rot or fire.
  - Example: "I sometimes get the smell of rotten fish inside my house."
- **Gustatory:** Experiencing tastes without any stimulus, often described as metallic or poisonous.
  - Example: "Whatever I eat, tastes like metal."
- **Cenesthetic:** Feeling bizarre sensations inside the body.
  - Example: "I can feel my organs shifting around or electricity running through my veins."
- **Kinesthetic:** A false perception of movement or of body parts being in a different position.
  - Example: "It feels like my arm is floating above my head, even though I can see it's right here beside me."

Schizophrenia

Schizophrenia is a severe and chronic mental disorder that causes significant disruptions in a person's thoughts, emotions, and behaviors, often leading to a detachment from reality.

Symptom Domains of Schizophrenia

Ophrenia is a complex mental disorder characterized by a range of symptoms across Schizophrenia is a complex mental disorder characterized by a range of symptoms across several domains (Fig. 2). **Positive symptoms** refer to the addition of new symptoms or an excess of normal functions. Examples include hallucinations, such as hearing voices (auditory hallucinations), and delusions, which are false, fixed beliefs not amenable to change, like believing one is a famous historical figure (grandiose delusion) or that others are plotting against them (paranoid delusion). **Negative symptoms** involve a decrease or loss of normal functions. This can manifest as alogia (poverty of speech), avolition (lack of motivation to pursue goals), anhedonia (inability to experience pleasure), and affective flattening (reduced emotional expression). **Cognitive symptoms** impact thinking, memory, and executive functions. Individuals might experience difficulty with attention and concentration, impaired working memory (e.g., struggling to remember instructions), and deficits in executive function, leading to poor problem-solving or planning. **Affective symptoms** relate to emotional dysregulation. These can include severe mood disturbances like depression, anxiety, mania, or inappropriate affect (e.g., laughing at a sad event). Finally, **aggressive symptoms** can involve agitation, hostility, and sometimes violent behavior, which may arise from paranoid delusions or command hallucinations.

While the symptoms in Fig. 2 can be present in many psychotic disorders, their combination and duration define the specific diagnosis. For instance, delusional disorder is characterized by one or more delusions for at least one month, but without the other prominent positive or negative symptoms of schizophrenia. Brief psychotic disorder involves the sudden onset of at least one positive symptom that lasts from one day to one month, with a full return to premorbid functioning. Schizoaffective

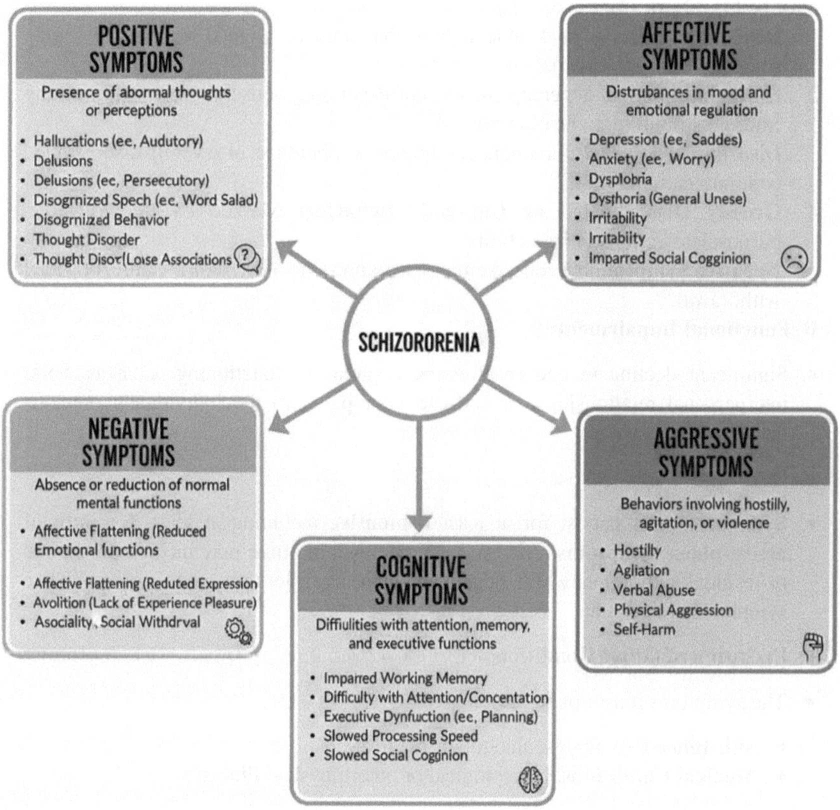

Fig. 2 The five symptom domains of Schizophrenia

disorder is diagnosed when a major mood episode (depressive or manic) occurs concurrently with the active-phase symptoms of schizophrenia, and delusions or hallucinations are also present for at least two weeks without a major mood episode.

Diagnosis of Schizophrenia

Schizophrenia is diagnosed based on the presence of specific symptoms and functional impairments, according to the DSM-5 (See Box 3).

Box 3 DSM-5 Diagnostic Criteria for Schizophrenia

A. Core Symptoms

Two or more of the following symptoms must be present for a significant portion of time during a **1-month period** (or less if successfully treated). At least one symptom must be (1), (2), or (3):

1. **Delusions:** False, unshakeable beliefs that are not aligned with reality (e.g., someone trying to harm).
2. **Hallucinations:** is a percept to the corresponding sensory organ without any external stimuli (e.g., hearing voices).
3. **Disorganized Speech:** Frequent derailment, incoherence, or severely disorganized communication.
4. **Grossly Disorganized or Catatonic Behavior:** Marked by unpredictable, purposeless actions or immobility.
5. **Negative Symptoms:** Reduced emotional expression, lack of motivation, or social withdrawal.

B. Functional Impairment

- Significant decline in one or more major areas of functioning, such as work, interpersonal relationships, or self-care, compared to the individual's previous levels.

C. Duration

- Symptoms must persist for at least **6 months**, including at least **1 month of active-phase symptoms** (criteria A). The remaining time may include prodromal or residual symptoms, where negative symptoms or less severe forms of positive symptoms are present.

D. Exclusion of Other Conditions

- The symptoms must not be attributable to:
  - **Substance Use**: Drugs, alcohol, or medications.
  - **Medical Conditions**: Neurological or other physical illnesses.

E. Schizoaffective Disorder and Mood Disorder Exclusion

- Schizoaffective disorder, depressive, or bipolar disorders with psychotic features must be ruled out. This is done by ensuring that mood symptoms are either absent or present only during a minority of the illness duration.

F. Developmental Disorders Exclusion

- If a history of autism spectrum disorder (ASD) or a communication disorder exists, schizophrenia is diagnosed only if prominent delusions or hallucinations are present for at least 1 month.

Other Psychotic Disorders

Apart from schizophrenia, the DSM-5 recognizes several other psychotic disorders, each with distinct criteria and features (Box 4). It is crucial to differentiate schizophrenia from other psychotic disorders, as treatment and prognosis can vary significantly.

Box 4 DSM-5 Diagnostic Criteria for Other Psychotic Disorders

1. **Schizoaffective Disorder**
   - **Definition:** A disorder that combines symptoms of schizophrenia (e.g., delusions, hallucinations) with a major mood episode (depressive or manic).
   - **Key Features:**
     - Psychotic symptoms (e.g., hallucinations or delusions) occur **independently** of mood symptoms for at least 2 weeks.
     - Mood episodes are prominent and last for the majority of the illness duration.
2. **Brief Psychotic Disorder**
   - **Definition:** A short-term psychotic disorder lasting **less than 1 month**, with eventual full recovery.
   - **Key Features:**
     - Presence of one or more core psychotic symptoms (delusions, hallucinations, disorganized speech, or disorganized behavior).
     - Triggered by stress, postpartum events, or no clear cause.
3. **Schizophreniform Disorder**
   - **Definition:** A psychotic disorder similar to schizophrenia but with symptoms lasting between 1 and 6 months.

- **Key Features:**
    - Symptoms meet the diagnostic criteria for schizophrenia, including functional impairments.
    - If symptoms persist beyond 6 months, the diagnosis may shift to schizophrenia.

4. **Delusional Disorder**

- **Definition:** A disorder characterized by the presence of **at least one type of delusions** lasting **1 month or longer**.
- **Key Features:**
    - Delusions are non-bizarre and involve situations that could occur in real life (e.g., being followed, loved, or persecuted).
    - Functioning is generally not impaired apart from the impact of the delusions.
    - No significant hallucinations, disorganized speech, or behavior.

5. **Shared Psychotic Disorder (Folie À Deux)**

- **Definition:** A rare condition where a delusion is shared between two or more people who are in a close relationship.
- **Key Features:**
    - One dominant person develops the delusion, and the other(s) adopt it.
    - Often occurs in isolated social settings.
    - Bangladesh example: Rita-Mita

6. **Substance/Medication-Induced Psychotic Disorder**

- **Definition:** Psychosis caused by substance use, intoxication, withdrawal, or medication side effects.
- **Key Features:**
    - Symptoms include delusions and/or hallucinations.
    - Directly linked to substance use or medication.

7. **Psychotic Disorder Due to Another Medical Condition**

- **Definition:** Psychotic symptoms caused by a medical condition, such as brain injury, tumor, or neurological disorders.
- **Key Features:**
    - Delusions, hallucinations, or disorganized behavior attributable to the medical condition.

8. **Catatonia Associated with Another Mental Disorder**

- **Definition:** A state of abnormal motor behavior associated with psychotic, mood, or medical conditions.

- **Key Features:**
  - Symptoms include stupor, mutism, posturing, waxy flexibility, or excessive motor activity.

9. **Unspecified Schizophrenia Spectrum and Other Psychotic Disorders**
   - **Definition:** A diagnosis used when psychotic symptoms are present, but they do not meet the full criteria for a specific psychotic disorder.
   - **Key Features:**
     - Used when there is insufficient information to make a definitive diagnosis.

10. **Postpartum Psychosis**
    - **Definition:** A severe psychotic disorder that occurs shortly after childbirth.
    - **Key Features:**
      - Symptoms include delusions, hallucinations, confusion, and impaired judgment.
      - Often associated with mood instability or manic symptoms.

Epidemiology

Psychotic disorders, including schizophrenia, pose a significant global health challenge.

- **Schizophrenia:** Schizophrenia is a globally prevalent psychiatric disorder affecting approximately 0.3–0.7% of the population, with an annual incidence of 1.5–10 cases per 100,000 individuals and an estimated 24 million people living with the condition worldwide. Although often described as universally distributed, epidemiological studies reveal notable variations: incidence is higher in urban environments and among certain immigrant and minority groups, while developing countries tend to report lower prevalence and better outcomes. The disorder typically emerges in late adolescence or early adulthood, with men showing earlier onset (late teens to mid-20 s) and women later onset (late 20 s to early 30 s), including a secondary peak around menopause. Lifetime prevalence is similar across sexes, but men often experience more severe symptoms. Risk factors identified through epidemiological research include family history, genetic vulnerability, prenatal complications, cannabis use during adolescence, childhood trauma, and social adversity linked to migration and discrimination. These patterns underscore schizophrenia's complex interplay of genetic, neurodevelopmental, and socio-environmental determinants, shaping its distribution and clinical presentation across populations.
- **Schizoaffective disorder:** Schizoaffective disorder combines psychotic symptoms with major mood episodes. It is less common than schizophrenia, with a

prevalence of about 0.3–0.8% and accounts for 10–30% of inpatient admissions for functional psychosis. Its epidemiology shows higher rates in women—mainly due to the depressive subtype—while the bipolar subtype affects both genders equally. Onset typically occurs in early adulthood (mean age ~ 25), with men experiencing earlier onset, and no major racial or geographic differences have been observed. Risk factors include a family history of schizophrenia or bipolar disorder, genetic overlap between these conditions, advanced paternal age, childhood trauma, significant life stressors, prenatal complications, and substance use (especially cannabis). These demographic patterns and risk factors underscore the complex interplay of genetic and environmental influences shaping the disorder's occurrence and presentation.

- **Delusional disorder:** Delusional disorder is a rarer condition, with a prevalence of 0.05–0.1%. It is characterized by persistent, non-bizarre delusions without other major symptoms of schizophrenia. Its onset is typically later in life, and it appears slightly more common in women. Delusional disorder is a rare psychiatric condition with a lifetime prevalence of about 0.02% and an annual incidence of 0.7–3 cases per 100,000 individuals, accounting for roughly 1–2% of inpatient psychiatric admissions. Its onset typically occurs in middle to late adulthood, with a mean age around 40 years. Epidemiological patterns show a slight female predominance, particularly for erotomanic delusions, while men are more likely to present with persecutory delusions. Additional risk factors include being single, divorced, or widowed (especially among women), low socioeconomic status, recent immigration, and social isolation, highlighting the influence of demographic and social determinants on its occurrence.
- **Brief psychotic disorder:** Brief psychotic disorder is a short-lived condition lasting between one day and one month. It often has a sudden onset, with a lifetime prevalence estimated at about 0.05% and an annual incidence of roughly 4 per 100,000 people, accounting for only about 1% of first-episode psychosis cases at follow-up. Epidemiological data suggest higher rates in developing countries—up to ten times more common than in industrialized nations—and among populations exposed to extreme stress, such as refugees, immigrants, and individuals affected by disasters like the COVID-19 pandemic. The disorder occurs most frequently in early to mid-adulthood, shows a slight female predominance, and carries an elevated risk during the postpartum period (1–2 per 1,000 births). These patterns underscore the strong association between psychosocial stressors and the occurrence of brief psychotic disorder, despite diagnostic challenges that contribute to uncertainty in prevalence estimates.

Etiology and Risk Factors

Epidemiological research consistently highlights several environmental risk factors, such as higher incidence in urban areas compared to rural regions and increased vulnerability among certain migrant and ethnic minority groups, pointing to the role of social and environmental stressors. Schizophrenia's origins are understood as a multifaceted interaction between strong genetic predispositions—supported by high heritability estimates—and environmental influences, including perinatal complications, advanced paternal age, and adolescent cannabis use. Consequently, the epidemiology of schizophrenia is far from uniform; it reflects a complex interplay of genetic, neurodevelopmental, and socioenvironmental factors that shape its varying incidence and clinical presentation (Box 5).

Neurobiology

Our understanding of the neurobiology of psychosis is most advanced for schizophrenia, but the core theories are considered relevant across the spectrum. These disorders are understood as neurodevelopmental, resulting from a complex interaction of genetic vulnerability and environmental factors.

Dopamine Hypothesis: This theory posits that an **excess of dopamine** activity in the mesolimbic pathway contributes to positive symptoms (delusions, hallucinations), while a **deficit of dopamine** in the mesocortical pathway may contribute to negative and cognitive symptoms. Most antipsychotic medications work by blocking dopamine D2 receptors.

Other Neurotransmitters: Dysregulation of **glutamate** and **serotonin** is also crucial. These systems interact with dopamine pathways and are targets for newer antipsychotic medications, which may improve efficacy for negative symptoms and reduce side effects.

Box 5 Major Risk Factors for Schizophrenia

1. **Genetic Factors**
   - Family History: Having a first-degree relative (e.g., parent, sibling) with schizophrenia increases the risk significantly.
   - Twin Studies: Concordance rates are higher in identical twins (40–50%) compared to fraternal twins.
   - Specific Genes: Variants in genes like DISC1, NRG1, and COMT are associated with increased susceptibility.
2. **Neurobiological Factors**
   - Dopamine Dysregulation: Over-activity in dopamine pathways contributes to positive symptoms like hallucinations and delusions.
   - Brain Structure Abnormalities: Enlargement of ventricles, reduced gray matter, and cortical thinning are common findings.
   - Neurodevelopmental Abnormalities: Issues during prenatal or early brain development may predispose individuals to schizophrenia.

3. **Environmental Factors**
   - Prenatal Complications:
     - Maternal malnutrition or infections during pregnancy (e.g., influenza, rubella).
     - Exposure to toxins or stress during fetal development.
   - Obstetric Complications:
     - Birth trauma, low birth weight, or hypoxia.
4. **Psychosocial Factors**
   - **Childhood Adversity:**
     - Physical, emotional, or sexual abuse.
     - Neglect or parental separation.
   - **Stressful Life Events:**
     - High-stress environments or traumatic events can trigger psychosis in vulnerable individuals.
5. **Substance Use**
   - Cannabis Use:
     - Strongly linked to an increased risk of developing schizophrenia, especially in those with a genetic predisposition.
   - Other Drugs:
     - Use of amphetamines, cocaine, or hallucinogens can exacerbate symptoms or lead to psychosis.
6. **Sociocultural Factors**
   - Urban Living: Growing up or living in urban areas increases the risk compared to rural settings.
   - Immigration: Higher rates of schizophrenia in immigrants, possibly due to stress and social adversity.
   - Social Isolation: Lack of meaningful social connections can increase vulnerability.
7. **Age and Gender**
   - **Age of Onset:** Schizophrenia typically develops in late adolescence or early adulthood.
   - **Gender Differences:**
     - Men: Earlier onset (late teens to early 20 s) with more severe symptoms.
     - Women: Later onset (late 20 s to early 30 s), often with better outcomes.

8. **Epigenetic and Inflammatory Factors**
   - **Epigenetic Changes:** Environmental factors can alter gene expression, increasing the risk.
   - **Immune System Dysregulation:** Elevated inflammatory markers (e.g., cytokines) are often observed in individuals with schizophrenia.

Course and Prognosis

The course and prognosis vary significantly across the psychotic disorders (Box 6). The course of schizophrenia is variable, but it is typically chronic. The illness often follows a pattern of an initial psychotic episode in late adolescence or early adulthood, followed by periods of remission and relapse. While full recovery is uncommon, many individuals can achieve significant symptom control and lead meaningful, productive lives. Positive prognostic factors include female gender, good premorbid functioning, later age of onset, and minimal negative symptoms.

Box 6 Course and Prognosis of Psychotic Disorder

- **Schizophrenia:** Typically, a chronic course with periods of remission and relapse. Full recovery is uncommon, but significant symptom control and a meaningful life are achievable.
- **Brief Psychotic Disorder:** By definition, involves a full return to premorbid functioning within one month. The prognosis is excellent.
- **Schizophreniform Disorder:** About two-thirds of individuals will go on to develop schizophrenia or schizoaffective disorder; one-third will recover.
- **Schizoaffective Disorder:** The prognosis is generally better than for schizophrenia but worse than for mood disorders alone.
- **Delusional Disorder:** The course is variable. It can be chronic, but functional impairment is often less severe than in schizophrenia, as the delusions may be encapsulated.

Medical Management

Schizophrenia treatment aims to reduce symptoms, prevent relapse, and enhance patient functionality through pharmacological and non-pharmacological interventions (Box 7).

Box 7 Medical Management of Schizophrenia

1. **Pharmacological Management**

   A. **Antipsychotics (Mainstay of Treatment)**

   - First-Generation Antipsychotics (FGAs)**:** Haloperidol, Trifluoperazine, Chlorpromazine, Fluphenazine.
   - Second-Generation Antipsychotics (SGAs)**:** Risperidone, Olanzapine, Quetiapine, Clozapine (treatment-resistant cases).
   - Long-Acting Injectable Antipsychotics (LAIs): For poor adherence.

   Examples: Fluphenazine, Zuclopenthixol, Paliperidone.

   B. **Adjunctive Medications**

   - Mood Stabilizers: Lithium, Valproate (for mood symptoms).
   - Antidepressants: Sertraline, Fluoxetine (for depressive symptoms).
   - Benzodiazepines: Lorazepam (for agitation/anxiety).

2. **Electroconvulsive Therapy (ECT)**

   - Used in treatment-resistant schizophrenia or severe agitation.

3. **Psychosocial Interventions**

   - CBT for Psychosis (CBTp): Identifies and challenges distorted thoughts.
   - Family Therapy: Improves communication and family support.
   - Social Skills Training: Enhances interpersonal and daily living skills.
   - Supported Employment: Assists in workplace reintegration.

4. **Lifestyle and Supportive Measures**

   - Diet & Exercise: Manages metabolic risks from medications.
   - Smoking Cessation Programs: Addresses common nicotine dependence.
   - Peer Support Groups: Reduces isolation and promotes recovery.

5. **Hospitalization (if Necessary)**
   For acute psychosis.

   - severe agitation, or risk of harm to self/others.

6. **Regular Monitoring & Follow-Up**

   - Ensure **medication adherence** and **side effect management** (e.g., EPS, weight gain, metabolic syndrome).
   - **Early detection** of relapse signs to prevent worsening of symptoms.

Table 2 Common antipsychotics and key nursing considerations

Class/medication	Key side effects	Nursing considerations
First-Generation (FGA) Haloperidol, Chlorpromazine	Extrapyramidal Symptoms (EPS): Akathisia, dystonia, Parkinsonism. Tardive Dyskinesia (TD). Anticholinergic effects	Monitor for muscle stiffness, restlessness, and abnormal movements. Administer anticholinergic agents (e.g., Benztropine) as ordered for EPS
Second-Generation (SGA) Risperidone, Olanzapine, Quetiapine	Metabolic Syndrome: Weight gain, hyperglycemia, dyslipidemia. Sedation	Monitor weight, BMI, waist circumference, fasting blood glucose, and lipid profile regularly. Encourage diet and exercise
Clozapine (SGA)	Agranulocytosis (fatal). Myocarditis, sedation, sialorrhea (hypersalivation), metabolic effects	Mandatory weekly-to-fortnightly WBC monitoring for the first 6 months. Monitor for fever and sore throat

Nursing Considerations for Antipsychotics

Antipsychotics are the cornerstone of treatment for most psychotic disorders. The nurse's role includes medication administration, monitoring for efficacy and side effects, and providing education. Key nursing considerations for common antipsychotic medications are shown in Table 2.

Nursing Management

Nursing care for clients with schizophrenia is a dynamic process focused on safety, building a therapeutic alliance, managing symptoms, and promoting recovery (Box 8). Management is long-term and follows a recovery-oriented, multidisciplinary approach. The psychiatric nurse plays a central role in coordinating care, administering treatments, and providing psychosocial support tailored to the specific disorder.

Box 8 Nursing Management of Schizophrenia

1. **Assessment**
   - **Mental Health:** Evaluate thought disturbances, hallucinations, delusions, and affect.
   - **Physical Health:** Monitor medication side effects (EPS, metabolic syndrome) and overall health.

- **Risk Factors:** Assess for self-harm, aggression, or suicide risk.

2. **Establishing a Therapeutic Relationship**
   - Build trust with empathy and consistency.
   - Maintain professional boundaries.

3. **Ensuring Safety**
   - Remove hazards from the environment.
   - Use de-escalation techniques for agitation.
   - Provide close observation during psychotic episodes.

4. **Medication Administration & Monitoring**
   - Ensure adherence to antipsychotics (e.g., risperidone, olanzapine).
   - Educate about medication effects and side effects.
   - Monitor for adverse effects like tardive dyskinesia and agranulocytosis (clozapine).

5. **Managing Symptoms**
   - **Hallucinations:** Acknowledge experiences without reinforcing them.
   - **Delusions:** Avoid arguing, focus on emotions.
   - **Cognitive Issues:** Use clear, simple language.

6. **Encouraging Social Interaction**
   - Facilitate group therapy and family involvement.
   - Provide one-on-one interactions to reduce isolation.

7. **Enhancing Self-Care & Independence**
   - Assist with hygiene and ADLs during acute phases.
   - Encourage a structured daily routine.

8. **Patient & Family Education**
   - Teach about schizophrenia, symptoms, and treatments.
   - Promote coping strategies (journaling, relaxation).
   - Emphasize medication adherence.

9. **Relapse Prevention**
   - Educate on early warning signs (withdrawal, anxiety).
   - Encourage follow-up care and peer support.

10. **Evaluation**
    - Monitor symptom improvement and medication adherence.
    - Assess quality of life and social reintegration.

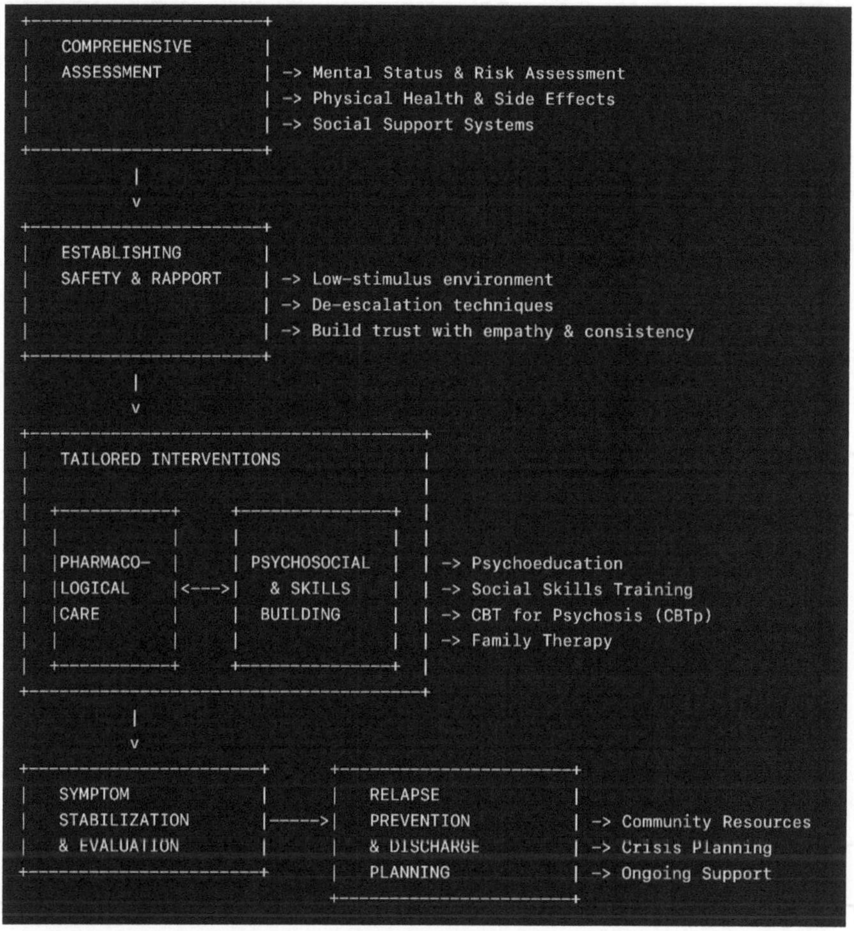

Fig. 3 Nursing management pathways of Schizophrenia

Nursing Management Pathway

The pathway of nursing management has been depicted in Fig. 3.

Nursing Assessment

A thorough nursing assessment is the foundation of care for any individual presenting with psychosis. It involves gathering information from multiple sources and performing a comprehensive examination to arrive at a provisional diagnosis and formulate a care plan (Boxes 7–9). Different psychometric tools could be useful (Box 10), and differential diagnoses should be carefully considered (Box 11).

Box 9 Principles of Nursing Assessment for Psychosis

- **Multiple Informants:** Always gather collateral information from family, carers, or previous healthcare providers, as the patient may lack insight into their illness.

  Examples:Haloperidol, Trifluoperazine, Chlorpromazine, Fluphenazine.
- **Safety First:** Assess for risk of harm to self or others, command hallucinations, and the ability to care for oneself.
- **Mental Status Examination (MSE):** A systematic evaluation of appearance, behaviour, speech, mood, affect, thought process, thought content, perception, cognition, and insight.
- **Physical Health Assessment:** Rule out medical causes of psychosis (e.g., delirium, thyroid dysfunction, substance intoxication) and establish a baseline for monitoring antipsychotic side effects (e.g., weight, blood pressure, blood glucose).

Box 10 Common Scales for Assessing Psychosis

- **Positive and Negative Syndrome Scale (PANSS):** A comprehensive, clinician-rated scale to measure symptom severity.
- **Brief Psychiatric Rating Scale (BPRS):** Widely used to assess a range of psychotic and mood symptoms.
- **Abnormal Involuntary Movement Scale (AIMS):** Used to screen for and monitor tardive dyskinesia, a potential side effect of antipsychotic medication.
- **Clinical Global Impression (CGI):** A brief scale used to rate the overall severity of illness and response to treatment.

Box 11 Differentiating Among Psychotic Disorders

- **Schizoaffective Disorder:** Characterized by the concurrent presence of symptoms of schizophrenia and a major mood episode (depressive or manic), with at least a 2-week period of delusions or hallucinations in the absence of a major mood episode.
- **Mood Disorder with Psychotic Features:** Psychotic symptoms occur exclusively during manic or depressive episodes.
- **Schizophreniform Disorder:** Identical symptoms to schizophrenia, but the duration is between 1 and 6 months.
- **Substance/Medication-Induced Psychotic Disorder:** Psychosis is a direct physiological consequence of a substance (e.g., cannabis, amphetamines, corticosteroids).
- **Psychosis due to Another Medical Condition:** Psychosis is caused by a medical illness, such as a brain tumor, delirium, or autoimmune encephalitis.

Table 3 Key areas of nursing interventions

Area	Interventions
Class/Medication Key Side Effects Nursing Considerations	Acknowledge the client's experience without reinforcing the delusion. Focus on the emotion: "I understand that hearing those voices is very frightening for you."
For Delusions	Avoid arguing or challenging the belief. Validate the underlying emotion: "It must feel very stressful to believe that you are being watched."
For Negative Symptoms:	Use a direct, supportive approach. Encourage small, achievable goals for self-care and social interaction. Provide structure and routine
Psychosocial	Administer antipsychotics as prescribed and monitor for side effects meticulously. Educate the client and family on the importance of adherence, even when feeling well
Medication Management & Education	Cannabis use (strongly linked, especially in adolescence), amphetamines, and cocaine

Key Areas of Nursing Interventions

Major areas of nursing interventions have been compared in Table 3.

Community Care and Relapse Prevention

The nurse's role is pivotal in preparing the client and family for discharge. Long-term management of schizophrenia occurs in the community. As a psychiatric nurse, providing advice to a patient with schizophrenia in the community helps them manage their condition, enhance quality of life, and prevent relapses (Box 12).

Box 12 Community Care of Schizophrenia

1. **Adherence to Treatment**
   - Take Medications as Prescribed: Never stop or skip medications without consulting your healthcare provider and report any side effects to your doctor for possible adjustments.
   - Attend Regular Check-Ups**:** Follow up with your psychiatrist or mental health professional regularly to monitor progress.
2. **Recognizing Early Warning Signs of Relapse**
   - Stay Alert for Symptoms: Identify early signs like increased anxiety, insomnia, withdrawal, or hearing voices.

- Seek Help Early: Contact your healthcare provider immediately if you notice these symptoms.

3. **Healthy Lifestyle Choices**
   - Eat a Balanced Diet: Include fruits, vegetables, whole grains, and proteins to maintain overall health.
   - Exercise Regularly: Engage in moderate physical activities like walking, yoga, or swimming to reduce stress.
   - Avoid Substances: Stay away from alcohol, drugs, and nicotine, as they can worsen symptoms or interfere with medications.

4. **Managing Stress**
   - Practice Relaxation Techniques: Use deep breathing, mindfulness, or meditation to cope with stress.
   - Follow a Routine: Create a structured daily schedule to provide stability and reduce confusion.
   - Take Breaks: Avoid overburdening yourself and take time for self-care.

5. **Building Social Connections**
   - Stay Connected: Engage with family and friends to avoid isolation.
   - Join Support Groups: Participate in local or online schizophrenia support groups for shared experiences and encouragement.
   - Improve Communication Skills: Practice social skills to build meaningful relationships.

6. **Engage in Productive Activities**
   - Volunteer or Work Part-Time: If possible, find activities that give you a sense of purpose.
   - Pursue Hobbies: Engage in interests like art, music, or gardening to enhance self-esteem and focus.

7. **Educate Yourself About Schizophrenia**
   - Understand the Illness: Learn about the condition to better manage symptoms and treatment.
   - Involve Your Family: Share educational resources with your family to improve their understanding and support.

8. **Utilize Community Resources**
   - Access Mental Health Services: Use local clinics, counselors, or rehabilitation centers for ongoing support.
   - Financial Support: Seek assistance programs for medications or other necessities, if needed.
   - Crisis Hotlines: Keep emergency contacts handy for immediate help during a crisis.

9. **Focus on Personal Safety**
   - Avoid Triggers: Identify and minimize exposure to situations or people that worsen your symptoms.
   - Inform Trusted Individuals**:** Let family or close friends know how to support you in case of emergencies.
10. **Be Patient and Positive**
    - Take Recovery Step by Step: Understand that managing schizophrenia is a gradual process, and progress takes time.
    - Celebrate Small Wins: Acknowledge every improvement, no matter how small.
    - Stay Hopeful**:** Remember that with proper care and support, a fulfilling life is possible.

3 Family Education

It is important to educate families that psychosis is a biological brain disorder to reduce stigma and to teach them to spot relapse signs, understand the diagnosis, and connect with community resources for support (Box 13).

Box 13 Key Components of Family Education

- Explain that psychotic disorders are biological brain disorders, not a result of poor parenting or personal weakness. This helps reduce guilt and blame.
- Teach the family to recognize early warning signs of relapse and to create a relapse prevention plan.
- Explain the specific diagnosis and its likely course (e.g., distinguishing between a one-time episode and a chronic condition).
- Provide information on community resources, such as the National Alliance on Mental Illness (NAMI), for support and advocacy.

4 Conditions that Require Referral to a Specialist

A specialist referral is crucial for a first psychotic episode, treatment resistance, or severe medication side effects. It is also necessary for significant suicide/violence risk or complex co-occurring medical/substance use disorders (Box 14).

Box 14 Referral to Specialist

- First psychotic episode (requires specialist early intervention services).
- Treatment resistance (failure to respond to adequate trials of standard treatments).
- Presence of severe or unmanageable medication side effects.
- Significant risk of suicide or violence.
- Complex co-occurring substance use or medical disorders.

Take Home Points

Schizophrenia is a complex disorder affecting thought, emotion, and behavior presenting with various symptoms.

- Diagnosis is clinical criteria, and requires ruling out other medical and psychiatric causes.
- Etiology involves a complex interaction of genetic, neurobiological, and environmental risk factors.
- Antipsychotic medications are the cornerstone of treatment but require vigilant monitoring for side effects.
- Nursing care is holistic, focusing on safety, therapeutic communication, symptom management, and patient/family education.
- Successful long-term management relies on community integration, relapse prevention strategies, and a strong support system.

Sample Multiple Choice Questions (MCQ) and Sample Best Answer Question

Signs and Symptoms of Schizophrenia include-			Which is a common nursing problem for clients with schizophrenia?		
T	(a)	Hallucinations are common		(a)	Anxiety
F	(b)	All exhibit the same symptoms	✓	(b)	Noncompliance with medication
T	(c)	Delusions affect perception		(c)	Low self-esteem
F	(d)	Symptoms don't vary in severity		(d)	Over activity
T	(e)	Negative symptoms include withdrawal			

Sample Short Questions

1. What are the DSM 5 diagnostic criteria of schizophrenia?
2. What is schizophrenia, with its risk factors/etiology?
3. Write down the signs & symptoms of schizophrenia.

4. Define delusion and its types.
5. Define hallucination and its types.

Sample Essay Questions

1. Explain the medical management of schizophrenia.
2. As a psychiatric nurse, how will you manage a case of schizophrenia in your ward?
3. What advice will you give to a Schizophrenic Patient in the community?

Suggested Reading

Bsn, P. M., RN. (2024). 6 Schizophrenia nursing care plans. Nurseslabs. https://nurseslabs.com/schizophrenia-nursing-care-plans/

Calabrese, J., Al Khalili, Y., & Shaheen, K. (2023). Psychosis (Nursing). In *StatPearls*. StatPearls Publishing. https://www.ncbi.nlm.nih.gov/books/NBK568796/?report=reader

Hany, M., Rizvi, A. (2024). Schizophrenia. In *StatPearls*. StatPearls Publishing. https://www.ncbi.nlm.nih.gov/books/NBK539864/

Keepers, G. A., Fochtmann, L. J., Anzia, J. M., Benjamin, S., Lyness, J. M., & Mojtabai, R. (2020). The American Psychiatric Association practice guideline for the treatment of patients with Schizophrenia. *American Journal of Psychiatry, 177*(9), 868–872. https://doi.org/10.1176/appi.ajp.2020.177901

Open Resources for Nursing; Ernstmeyer, K., & Christman, E. (Eds.). (2022). *Nursing: Mental health and community concepts*. Eau Claire (WI): Chippewa Valley Technical College; 2022. Chapter 11 Psychosis and Schizophrenia. https://www.ncbi.nlm.nih.gov/books/NBK590027/

National Institute for Health and Care Excellence (NICE). (2014, March). Psychosis and schizophrenia in adults: Prevention and management (NICE Clinical Guidelines, No. 178). https://www.ncbi.nlm.nih.gov/books/NBK555203/

Chapter 6
Care of Clients with Mood Disorders

Bithika Mali and S. M. Yasir Arafat

Abstract Mood disorders encompass a range of psychiatric conditions such as major depressive disorder, bipolar I and II disorders, persistent depressive disorder (dysthymia), and cyclothymia, characterized by sustained disruptions in emotional regulation. This chapter delivers a comprehensive, nursing-focused examination of these disorders, covering diagnostic frameworks and their implications for tailored interventions. Taking a biopsychosocial perspective, it explores the multifactorial origins of mood disorders, including genetic predispositions, neurochemical imbalances, psychological vulnerabilities, and sociocultural stressors. Clinical manifestations across depressive, manic/hypomanic, and mixed states are described to support accurate assessment. Emphasis is placed on nursing assessment tools and strategies such as mental status examination and the use of validated scales, alongside holistic evaluations informed by the nursing process. Nursing interventions are outlined at each stage: acute stabilization, safety planning, psychoeducation, therapeutic communication, fostering routine and structure, collaboration with interdisciplinary teams, and relapse prevention. This chapter aims to equip nurses with evidence-based, person-centered approaches for managing mood disorders across diverse care settings.

Keywords Mood disorders · Major depressive disorder · Bipolar disorder · Classification · Etiology · Assessment · Management · Nursing · Psychoeducation

B. Mali
Department of Graduate Nursing, Bangladesh Medical University, Dhaka, Bangladesh

S. M. Y. Arafat (✉)
Department of Psychiatry, Bangladesh Specialized Hospital, Dhaka, Bangladesh
e-mail: arafatdmc62@gmail.com

S. M. Y. Arafat and H. Akter (eds.), *Psychiatric Nursing in Bangladesh*, Mental Health Systems and Policy in Low- and Middle-Income Countries,
https://doi.org/10.1007/978-981-95-8501-4_6

1 Introduction

Mood disorders, encompassing major depressive disorder, bipolar disorder, and related affective conditions, represent a considerable and growing public health concern worldwide. Their impact extends outside individual suffering to profound societal and economic costs. According to the World Health Organization (WHO), depression alone affects more than 280 million people globally, contributing significantly to the overall burden of disease and disability. In low- and middle-income countries, including Bangladesh, the prevalence and consequences of mood disorders are often neglected due to limited resources, stigma, and gaps in mental health infrastructure.

Bangladesh, a densely populated country in South Asia, has witnessed rising rates of depression and anxiety disorders over recent decades. Epidemiological studies suggest that approximately 6–7% of the Bangladeshi population is affected by depressive disorders, with higher prevalence observed among women and socioeconomically disadvantaged groups. Despite this burden, mental health services remain underdeveloped, with less than one psychiatrist per million people and limited access to evidence-based interventions. This context underscores the urgency of expanding the capacity of non-specialist health professionals, including nurses, to address mood disorders effectively.

Nurses play a pivotal role in the early detection, management, and rehabilitation of individuals living with mood disorders, especially in cases of comorbid and chronic depressive states. Positioned at the forefront of primary and community health care, nurses are often the first point of contact for patients and families. Their responsibilities encompass screening for symptoms, providing psychoeducation, delivering supportive counseling, monitoring treatment adherence, and coordinating multidisciplinary care. In Bangladesh and similar settings, empowering nurses with the knowledge and skills to manage mood disorders can bridge critical gaps in service delivery and improve health outcomes.

Definition

Mood

Mood is defined as a persistent, pervasive, and predominant emotional state that influences an individual's perception of the world, self, and environment. Unlike acute emotions, which are typically brief and reactive to specific stimuli, mood represents a more generalized affective tone that can persist for hours, days, or longer. It moderates thought processes, motivation, and behavior and is often described subjectively by individuals using terms such as sad, anxious, irritable, or euphoric.

Mood Disorders

Mood disorders are mental health conditions that cause strong changes in a person's mood, like long-lasting sadness or extreme happiness (mania), which affect daily life. Common mood disorders include major depression, bipolar disorder, persistent depressive disorder (dysthymia), and cyclothymia. These conditions can lead to problems with thinking, physical health, behavior, and social life. They often come with other illnesses and may increase the risk of disability or early death.

2 Classification of Mood Disorders

Mood disorders are classified within established diagnostic frameworks, principally the *International Classification of Diseases*, 11th Revision (ICD-11) and the *Diagnostic and Statistical Manual of Mental Disorders, Fifth Edition* (DSM-5, Box 1).

ICD-11 Classification

In the ICD-11, mood disorders are grouped under *Mood Disorders (6A60–6A8Z)*, with key categories:

- Depressive disorders (e.g., single/recurrent depressive disorder)
- Bipolar disorders (e.g., bipolar I & II)
- Persistent mood disorders (e.g., dysthymia, cyclothymia)
- Other/unspecified mood disorders

DSM-5 Classification

The DSM-5 divides mood disorders into two main groups:

- Depressive Disorders
- Bipolar and Related Disorders

This separation reflects growing evidence that depressive and bipolar conditions represent distinct clusters in terms of symptom patterns, longitudinal course, and treatment response.

Depressive Disorders

Depressive disorders are characterized by sustained low mood, diminished interest or pleasure, and cognitive and somatic symptoms. Key diagnoses include:

- Major Depressive Disorder (MDD)
- Persistent Depressive Disorder (Dysthymia)

- Disruptive Mood Dysregulation Disorder (in children and adolescents)
- Premenstrual Dysphoric Disorder

Bipolar Disorders

Bipolar disorders involve episodes of mania or hypomania alternating with depressive episodes. The primary subtypes are:

- Bipolar I Disorder (at least one manic episode, typically with depressive episodes)
- Bipolar II Disorder (at least one hypomanic episode and one major depressive episode)
- Cyclothymic Disorder (chronic fluctuating mood disturbances with subthreshold hypomanic and depressive symptoms)

Persistent Mood Disorders

Persistent mood disorders, such as dysthymia and cyclothymia, are characterized by chronic, less severe mood disturbances lasting for years. Though symptoms may be milder than those of episodic mood disorders, their long duration often leads to significant impairment.

Mixed Affective States

Mixed affective states refer to episodes in which features of both mania/hypomania and depression occur simultaneously or in rapid alternation. DSM-5 includes *"with mixed features"* specifiers for both depressive and manic episodes, acknowledging the frequent overlap of mood symptoms that do not fit neatly into categorical definitions. Recognition of mixed presentations is clinically important, as they are associated with higher symptom burden, increased suicidality, and more complex treatment needs.

Box 1. Classification of Mood Disorders

ICD-11 Classification

- Depressive disorders (e.g., single/recurrent depressive disorder)
- Bipolar or related disorders (e.g., bipolar type I and II disorder)
- Persistent mood disorders (e.g., dysthymia, cyclothymia)
- Other specified or unspecified mood disorders

DSM-5 Classification

- Depressive Disorders
- Bipolar and Related Disorders

Depressive Disorders

Include low mood, loss of interest, fatigue, and poor concentration:

- Major Depressive Disorder (MDD)
- Persistent Depressive Disorder (Dysthymia)
- Disruptive Mood Dysregulation Disorder (in children and adolescents)
- Premenstrual Dysphoric Disorder

Bipolar Disorders

Involve mood swings between mania/hypomania and depression:

- Bipolar I (manic ± depressive episodes)
- Bipolar II (hypomanic + depressive episodes)
- Cyclothymic Disorder (mild, chronic mood swings

Persistent Mood Disorders

- Chronic, less severe but long-lasting mood disturbances like dysthymia and cyclothymia

Mixed Affective States

- Mixed affective states refer to episodes in which features of both mania/hypomania and depression occur simultaneously or in rapid alternation.

Clinical Manifestations of Mood Disorders

Mood disorders present with a range of emotional, cognitive, behavioral, and physical symptoms (Table 1). The clinical features differ depending on the predominant mood state, whether depressive or manic, and the severity and duration of episodes.

Table 1 Clinical features of mood disorders

Depression	Mania/Hypomania
• Low mood • Loss of interest or pleasure in most activities • Fatigue or low energy • Sleep disturbances (insomnia or hypersomnia) • Changes in appetite or weight • Psychomotor agitation or retardation • Feelings of worthlessness or guilt • Poor concentration or indecisiveness • Suicidal thoughts • Persistent sadness, hopelessness, or emptiness	• Elevated, expansive, or irritable mood • Inflated self-esteem or grandiosity • Decreased need for sleep • Increased talkativeness • Racing thoughts or flight of ideas • Distractibility • Heightened goal-directed activity • Risky or impulsive behaviors

Depression: Signs and Symptoms

According to the DSM-5, diagnosing a major depressive episode requires at least five of nine symptoms to be present for most of the day, nearly every day, for at least two weeks.

Here are the nine symptoms listed in the DSM-5 for a major depressive episode:

1. **Depressed Mood:** This can be a subjective feeling of sadness, emptiness, or hopelessness, or it can be observed by others, such as appearing tearful. In children and adolescents, this may present as an irritable mood.
2. **Loss of Interest or Pleasure:** A markedly diminished interest or pleasure in most or all normal activities, which may be reported by the individual or observed by others.
3. **Weight and Appetite Changes:** Significant weight loss (when not dieting) or gain, or a decrease or increase in appetite nearly every day. For children, this may be a failure to make expected weight gains.
4. **Sleep Disturbance:** Insomnia or hypersomnia (sleeping too much) nearly every day.
5. **Psychomotor Changes:** Psychomotor agitation (restlessness) or retardation (slowed movements or speech) that is noticeable to others.
6. **Fatigue or Loss of Energy:** Feeling tired or having a general lack of energy, making routine tasks difficult.
7. **Feelings of Worthlessness or Guilt:** Excessive or inappropriate feelings of worthlessness or guilt that may be delusional, and not simply self-reproach for being sick.
8. **Impaired Concentration:** A diminished ability to think, concentrate, or make decisions, reported subjectively or observed by others.
9. **Recurrent Thoughts of Death or Suicide:** Recurrent thoughts of death, suicidal ideation (without a specific plan), a suicide attempt, or a specific plan for suicide. These symptoms must be present most of the day, nearly every day, for at least two weeks to meet diagnostic criteria for a major depressive episode.

Mania and Hypomania: Signs and Symptoms

According to the DSM-5, both mania and hypomania involve symptoms like elevated mood, increased energy, less need for sleep, rapid speech, racing thoughts, distractibility, goal-directed activity, and risky behaviors. The key differences are the duration and severity: mania requires symptoms for at least one week (or any duration if hospitalization is needed) and causes significant impairment in functioning or psychosis, while hypomania requires symptoms for at least four days and does not cause severe impairment or psychosis.

Core Symptoms (for Both Mania and Hypomania)

An individual must experience a distinct period of abnormally and persistently elevated, expansive, or irritable mood and increased activity or energy. During this period, at least three of the following symptoms must be present (four if the mood is only irritable):

- **Inflated self-esteem or grandiosity**: A sense of exaggerated self-importance.
- **Decreased need for sleep**: Feeling rested after only a few hours of sleep.
- **More talkative than usual or pressured to keep talking**: Talking rapidly and at an unusually high volume.
- **Flight of ideas or racing thoughts**: Subjective experience of thoughts moving quickly from one idea to another.
- **Distractibility**: Attention is too easily drawn to unimportant or irrelevant external stimuli.
- **Increase in goal-directed activity**: Engaging in more goal-focused behavior at work, school, or socially.
- **Psychomotor agitation**: Purposeless, non-goal-directed physical activity.
- **Excessive involvement in pleasurable activities**: Engaging in activities that have a high potential for painful consequences, such as unrestrained buying sprees, sexual indiscretions, or foolish business investments.

Suicide Risk Indicators

Mood disorders are strongly associated with increased risk of suicide. Clinicians should be alert for warning signs, including:

- Expressed or implied suicidal thoughts or plans
- Previous suicide attempts or self-harm behaviors
- Severe hopelessness or feelings of worthlessness
- Marked agitation or anxiety
- Abrupt withdrawal from social relationships
- Sudden improvement in mood after a depressive episode (which may signal intent to act)
- Access to means of self-harm

Routine risk assessment and safety planning are essential components of care for individuals with mood disorders, particularly during acute depressive or mixed affective states.

3 Etiology/Risk Factors of Mood Disorders

The development of mood disorders is multifactorial, arising from complex interactions among biological, psychological, social, and cultural determinants. Understanding these factors is essential for effective prevention, assessment, and intervention.

Biological Factors

Genetic predisposition plays a significant role in the etiology of mood disorders. Family and twin studies have consistently demonstrated higher rates of major depressive disorder and bipolar disorder among first-degree relatives of affected individuals. Heritability estimates are approximately 40–50% for major depressive disorder and up to 80% for bipolar disorder, suggesting a strong genetic contribution, particularly in bipolar syndromes.

Neurobiological mechanisms also reinforce mood disorders. Dysregulation of monoamine neurotransmitters, including serotonin, norepinephrine, and dopamine, is implicated in the pathophysiology of depression. Abnormalities in glutamatergic transmission and neuroplasticity have further been identified as potential contributors. In bipolar disorder, alterations in circadian rhythms and cellular signaling pathways are also believed to influence mood instability.

Psychological Factors

Certain personality traits and psychological vulnerabilities can increase susceptibility to mood disorders. High levels of neuroticism, low self-esteem, and maladaptive coping styles have been associated with an elevated risk of depression. Early life adversity, such as childhood trauma, abuse, or neglect, can disrupt emotional regulation and heighten sensitivity to stress later in life. Traumatic experiences, particularly those involving loss or interpersonal violence, are powerful triggers for mood symptoms.

Social Factors

Social determinants play a critical role in the onset and course of mood disorders. Poverty, economic insecurity, and chronic life stressors contribute to increased psychological distress and reduced access to mental health services. Dysfunctional family dynamics, including conflict, overprotection, or lack of support, have been linked to higher rates of depressive episodes and poor outcomes. Social isolation and lack of meaningful community connections can further multiple vulnerabilities.

Cultural Considerations

Cultural, economic, and structural factors uniquely shape the experience and expression of mood disorders. Persistent poverty, rapid urbanization, and political instability create chronic stress that increases mental health risks (Box 2). Cultural stigma surrounding mental illness often discourages individuals from seeking help, leading to delays in diagnosis and treatment.

Box 2. Risk Factors of Mood Disorders

- Biological: Genetic vulnerability is significant, with heritability up to 50% in depression and 80% in bipolar disorder. Neurotransmitter imbalances (serotonin, norepinephrine, and dopamine) and circadian rhythm disruptions also contribute.
- Psychological: Traits such as neuroticism, low self-esteem, and maladaptive coping increase risk. Early trauma, abuse, and loss are strong predictors of later mood disturbances.
- Social: Poverty, chronic stress, family conflict, and social isolation are key environmental stressors that heighten vulnerability and hinder recovery.

Cultural: High stigma, somatic presentations of symptoms, limited mental health services, and the influence of religious and family norms shape the experience and treatment of mood disorders. Persistent poverty and rapid urbanization further exacerbate mental health risks.

4 Assessment and Diagnosis

Diagnosis of Mood Disorders

Accurate diagnosis of mood disorders is foundational to effective treatment and management. Diagnostic criteria, validated assessment tools, and comprehensive clinical evaluation together guide health professionals in identifying mood disorders and differentiating them from other psychiatric or medical conditions.

DSM-5 Criteria

The DSM-5 remains the standard reference for diagnosing mood disorders. It outlines specific criteria for major depressive disorder, bipolar I and II disorders, persistent depressive disorder, and other related conditions. Diagnosis requires the presence of characteristic symptom clusters over defined durations, e.g., at least two weeks of depressed mood or anhedonia accompanied by cognitive and somatic symptoms for major depressive disorder. Bipolar disorders necessitate distinct manic or hypomanic episodes, defined by elevated mood and increased activity lasting at least four consecutive days (hypomania) or seven days (mania), with associated functional impairment. The DSM-5 further allows for the use of specifiers, such as severity, presence of psychotic features, and mixed features, to refine diagnosis and inform treatment planning.

Assessment Tools

In clinical practice, structured screening instruments supplement diagnostic interviews by providing standardized measures of symptom severity and assisting in early identification. Two widely used tools are:

- **Patient Health Questionnaire-9 (PHQ-9):** A brief, self-administered scale assessing the frequency of nine depressive symptoms over the past two weeks. It provides a quantitative measure of depression severity and is validated for use in diverse populations.
- **Mood Disorder Questionnaire (MDQ):** A screening tool designed to detect bipolar disorder by querying the lifetime history of manic or hypomanic symptoms. The MDQ helps differentiate bipolar disorder from unipolar depression, facilitating timely referral and intervention.

Nursing Role in Assessment

Nurses play an integral role in the diagnostic process, particularly in settings where they serve as frontline healthcare providers. Their responsibilities include:

- Administering and interpreting screening tools such as PHQ-9 and MDQ
- Conducting thorough clinical interviews to elicit symptom history, functional impact, and psychosocial context
- Observing behavioral and affective signs during patient interactions
- Identifying risk factors and warning signs of suicidality or worsening symptoms
- Coordinating multidisciplinary evaluations and communicating findings to mental health specialists

The nursing assessment provides critical data that informs diagnosis, treatment planning, and ongoing monitoring.

Medical Management of Mood Disorders

The treatment of mood disorders necessitates a comprehensive, multidisciplinary approach encompassing pharmacological, somatic, and psychotherapeutic interventions tailored to the specific diagnosis and individual patient needs (Box 3). In resource-limited settings such as Bangladesh, adapting evidence-based treatments within cultural and systemic constraints remains a clinical priority. In some cases, mood disorders are best addressed with medication. Medication can be extremely important in managing mood disorder symptoms, but this also requires close monitoring by a healthcare provider. Some clients may need to try different medications before their physician finds the one that works best.

Pharmacological Treatments

Pharmacotherapy is a cornerstone in managing mood disorders.

- **Antidepressants** are primarily indicated for depressive episodes. Selective serotonin reuptake inhibitors (SSRIs) are the first-line agents due to their favorable safety profile and tolerability. Other classes include serotonin-norepinephrine reuptake inhibitors (SNRIs), tricyclic antidepressants (TCAs), and monoamine oxidase inhibitors (MAOIs), though the latter are less commonly used due to side effects and dietary restrictions.
- **Mood stabilizers**, such as lithium and anticonvulsants (e.g., valproate, carbamazepine), are essential for bipolar disorder to control manic and depressive episodes and reduce relapse risk. Lithium remains the gold standard for long-term mood stabilization and suicide prevention, but requires regular monitoring of serum levels and renal function.
- **Antipsychotics**, particularly second-generation (atypical) agents like quetiapine and olanzapine, are employed to manage acute mania, mixed episodes, and as adjuncts in treatment-resistant depression. Their use must be balanced against metabolic and extrapyramidal side effects.
- **Anxiolytic medications:** Also called anti-anxiety medications, they are designed to lower anxiety and can be used to treat social anxiety, panic disorder, and other anxiety-related illnesses.

Electroconvulsive Therapy (ECT)

ECT is an effective somatic treatment for severe, treatment-resistant mood disorders, especially major depression with psychotic features, catatonia, or suicidal risk. In Bangladesh, ECT is practiced predominantly in tertiary centers and psychiatric hospitals due to limited infrastructure and stigma associated with the procedure. Despite these challenges, ECT remains a vital option given its rapid efficacy and safety profile when administered with modern anesthesia and muscle relaxants.

Psychotherapies

Psychotherapeutic modalities complement pharmacotherapy and are crucial in relapse prevention and functional recovery.

- **Cognitive Behavioral Therapy (CBT)** focuses on identifying and modifying negative thought patterns and behaviors contributing to mood symptoms. It has demonstrated efficacy in both depressive and bipolar disorders.
- **Interpersonal Therapy (IPT)** addresses interpersonal issues and role transitions that may trigger mood episodes. IPT is particularly effective in depression and is adaptable to diverse cultural contexts.

Lifestyle Modifications and Psychoeducation

Lifestyle interventions, including regular physical activity, sleep hygiene, and stress management, support overall mental health and treatment adherence. Psychoeducation for patients and families enhances understanding of the illness, promotes medication compliance, and facilitates early recognition of relapse signs. In Bangladesh, culturally sensitive psychoeducation is vital to overcome stigma and engage community and family resources in care.

There are many modifications people can make to their lifestyle and daily routines that can make life easier for those living with bipolar. Recognizing that each person's experience is unique, a variety of tips are presented that can be applied to your life.

Some lifestyle modifications to help cope with mood disorders include:

- Develop a sleep schedule: Both the body and brain need rest, and sleep hygiene may be effective in helping improve mood.
- Daily exercise: Regular exercise has been shown to be effective in improving mood, so add a daily walk, at the least, to your routine.
- Adopt a regular schedule for meals: A consistent routine acts as a reminder to keep moving during the day and helps balance out your body's schedule.
- Increase intake of fresh vegetables and fruits: These fresh foods can offer protection against anxiety and depression due to the nutrients they pack.

- Integrate mindfulness into your life: Mindfulness and breathwork are able to calm the body through lowering blood pressure, decreasing cortisol levels, and lowering the heart rate.
- Spend time outside every day: Exposure to green space and nature is also effective in positively influencing our overall well-being. It decreases health risks as it boosts our moods.
- Abstain from alcohol: This is especially true if you are on medication, but trying to self-medicate mood disorders with alcohol is counterproductive. Alcohol is a depressant, and it also interrupts sleep.
- Keep a journal/mood diary**:** A journaling practice encourages you to write about what's going on inside, as well as provides a tracking system so that you can determine if there are certain events, people, or situations that trigger manic or depressive episodes.

Box 3. Medical Management of Mood Disorders

Pharmacological Treatments ÷

- Antidepressants (SSRIs, SNRIs, TCAs) for depressive episodes.
- Mood stabilizers (lithium, valproate, carbamazepine) for bipolar disorder.
- Antipsychotics (atypical agents like quetiapine, olanzapine) for mania and adjunctive therapy.
- Anxiolytic medications are used to treat social anxiety, panic disorder, and other anxiety-related illnesses.

Electroconvulsive Therapy (ECT) ÷

- Used for severe, treatment-resistant mood disorders.
- Available in tertiary centers in Bangladesh.
- Effective and rapid, especially for psychotic depression and suicidal risk.

Psychotherapies ÷

- Cognitive Behavioral Therapy (CBT) targets negative thoughts and behaviors.
- Interpersonal Therapy (IPT) addresses interpersonal triggers and role transitions.

Lifestyle and Psychoeducation ÷

- Emphasizes physical activity, sleep hygiene, and stress management.
- Psychoeducation improves medication adherence and relapse prevention.
- Cultural sensitivity is important in Bangladesh to reduce stigma and engage families.

Nursing Management of Mood Disorders

Nursing care is central to the comprehensive management of mood disorders. Through systematic assessment, individualized care planning, and therapeutic engagement, nurses help alleviate symptoms, promote safety, and support recovery (Box 4). In Bangladesh, nursing interventions must be adapted to available resources, cultural expectations, and family dynamics.

Common Nursing Diagnoses

Patients with mood disorders may present with diverse needs that guide nursing diagnoses. Common examples include:

- Medication compliance
- Risk for suicide is related to hopelessness and depressed mood
- Disturbed sleep pattern related to mood disturbance
- Ineffective coping related to inadequate support systems
- Self-care deficit related to low energy and lack of motivation
- Social isolation is related to withdrawal and anhedonia
- Imbalanced nutrition related to decreased appetite or excessive eating

Nursing Care Plan

Developing an effective nursing care plan requires culturally sensitive, realistic goals. Key components include:

- **Assessment:** Ongoing monitoring of mood, behavior, thought content (including suicidal ideation), sleep, appetite, and functioning. In Bangladesh, nurses often rely on both patient reports and input from family members due to cultural emphasis on family caregiving.
- **Planning and Implementation**
    - Establish structured daily routines to support sleep and self-care.
    - Provide psychoeducation to patients and families about symptom management and treatment adherence.
    - Facilitate referrals to community health workers and mental health resources when available.
    - Encourage participation in culturally acceptable social and spiritual supports.
- **Evaluation:** Regular review of progress toward goals, symptom reduction, and functional improvement.

Communication and Therapeutic Relationship

Establishing trust is fundamental in caring for individuals with mood disorders. Therapeutic communication principles include:

- Active listening and nonjudgmental acceptance of feelings
- Using simple, clear language to convey information
- Allowing time for response, particularly when psychomotor slowing is present
- Validating emotions while fostering hope and engagement
- Maintaining appropriate professional boundaries

In Bangladesh, cultural respect and involving family decision-makers are important to build rapport and encourage adherence.

Safety Precautions

Ensuring patient safety is a priority, especially when there is risk of self-harm or suicide. Precautions may include:

- Close observation or suicide watch as indicated
- Removal of potentially harmful objects from the environment
- Frequent reassessment of suicidal thoughts

Box 4. Nursing Management of Mood Disorders

Common Nursing Diagnoses

- Risk for suicide is related to hopelessness and mood disturbance.
- Disturbed thought processes related to biochemical alterations.
- Self-care deficit related to decreased energy and motivation.
- Ineffective coping is related to a maladaptive stress response.

Nursing Care Plan

- Prioritize safety and suicide prevention.
- Monitor mood, behavior, and medication adherence.
- Educate patients and families about illness, treatment, and relapse signs.
- Collaborate with community resources and address cultural stigma.

Communication and Therapeutic Relationship

- Use empathetic, nonjudgmental listening.
- Establish trust through consistency and respect.
- Encourage expression of feelings without fear of criticism.

Safety Precautions

- Implement suicide watch if indicated.
- Restrict access to harmful objects and medications.
- Ensure environmental safety and close observation during crises.

Nursing Interventions

1. **Risk Management**
    - Conduct frequent suicide risk assessments; implement suicide precautions if necessary.
    - Remove potentially harmful objects from the patient's environment.
    - Maintain close observation and ensure safety protocols.
2. **Emotional Support and Therapeutic Communication**
    - Establish trust through active listening, empathy, and validation of feelings.
    - Encourage verbalization of emotions and fears.
    - Provide a consistent, nonjudgmental presence to reduce isolation.
3. **Promoting Coping and Self-Care**
    - Teach and reinforce adaptive coping techniques (e.g., relaxation exercises, journaling).
    - Assist with personal hygiene and nutrition as needed, gradually encouraging independence.
    - Facilitate participation in structured daily activities and social interactions.
4. **Psychoeducation**
    - Educate the patient and family about the nature of mood disorders, treatment plans, and the importance of medication adherence.
    - Discuss early warning signs of relapse and emergency contacts.
    - Address cultural beliefs and stigma to promote understanding and acceptance.
5. **Coordination of Care**
    - Collaborate with psychiatrists for medication management.
    - Refer to counseling or psychotherapy services (CBT or IPT).
    - Link the family with community support groups as appropriate.

5 Patient and Family Education of Mood Disorders

Patient and family education is a fundamental component of effective management and long-term recovery in mood disorders. Comprehensive psychoeducation empowers individuals to understand their illness, adhere to treatment, and engage supportive networks that promote stability and well-being (Box 5).

Treatment Adherence

Education on treatment adherence emphasizes the importance of taking medications consistently, attending scheduled appointments, and following therapeutic recommendations. Nurses should explain:

- The purpose and expected benefits of prescribed medications, such as antidepressants, mood stabilizers, or antipsychotics.
- Potential side effects and strategies to manage them.
- The risks associated with abrupt discontinuation or irregular dosing include symptom recurrence and withdrawal effects.
- The need for regular monitoring, such as blood tests for lithium therapy or metabolic screening for antipsychotics.

Relapse Prevention

Patients and families should be educated to recognize early warning signs of relapse, including subtle mood changes, sleep disturbances, decreased motivation, or irritability. Education should cover:

- Developing a personalized relapse prevention plan outlining specific symptoms to watch for and steps to take when early signs appear.
- The importance of maintaining regular routines, adequate sleep, and healthy coping strategies.
- Strategies for managing stress and identifying triggers that may precipitate episodes.

Involving family members in planning enhances vigilance and timely intervention.

Support Systems

Education should highlight the role of support systems in sustaining recovery. Nurses can guide patients and families to:

- Identify and engage trusted family members, friends, or community resources who can provide practical and emotional support.
- Utilize available mental health services, including counseling and community mental health programs.
- Participate in peer support groups or advocacy networks that promote shared learning and reduce isolation.

Encouraging open communication within families helps create an environment of understanding and acceptance, which is particularly important in cultures where mental health stigma persists.

Box 5. Patient and Family Education of Mood Disorders

Treatment Adherence

- Explain the purpose, benefits, and side effects of medications.
- Emphasize the importance of regular dosing and follow-up visits.
- Address misconceptions and stigma sensitively, especially in Bangladesh.

Relapse Prevention

- Teach recognition of early warning signs (e.g., mood changes, sleep issues).
- Develop individualized relapse prevention plans.
- Encourage healthy routines and stress management strategies.

Support Systems

- Identify trusted family, friends, and community resources.
- Promote use of mental health services and peer support groups.
- Foster open communication and understanding within the family.

Take Home Messages

- Mood disorders involve persistent emotional disturbances (e.g., depression, bipolar disorder).
- Major types: MDD, Bipolar I/II, Persistent Depressive Disorder.
- High stigma leads to underreporting; patients often present with somatic symptoms (e.g., fatigue, pain).
- Family involvement is critical due to collective societal structures.
- Safety first: Always assess suicide risk.
- Use culturally adapted tools (e.g., Bengali PHQ-9).
- Educate families to combat myths (e.g., "possession" beliefs).
- Medications: SSRIs (depression), mood stabilizers (bipolar).
- Therapies: CBT, family therapy, and integrative care (e.g., spiritual support).
- Limited mental health resources; nurses often bridge gaps between traditional healers and medical care.
- Therapeutic communication that respects cultural/religious beliefs while promoting evidence-based care.

Sample Short Answer Questions

1. What are the key differences between a manic episode and a depressive episode in bipolar disorder?
2. How would you assess suicide risk in a Bangladeshi patient?

Sample Essay Questions

1. Discuss the bio-psycho-social-spiritual model of mood disorders with examples.
2. Describe the classification of mood disorders.
3. Describe the role of a nurse in managing a bipolar disorder patient in your ward.
4. What nursing interventions are essential for a manic patient?

1. Which neurotransmitter imbalance is most associated with Major Depressive Disorder (MDD)?			2. All patients with Major Depressive Disorder (MDD) require hospitalization		
	(a)	Dopamine	T	(a)	Depression is always dangerous
✓	(b)	Low serotonin	F	(b)	Only suicidal cases need admission
	(c)	High GABA	T	(c)	24-h observation
	(d)	Acetylcholine deficiency	F	(d)	Most can be treated, outpatient
			T	(e)	Required by law in Bangladesh

Suggested Reading

Amin, M. T., Ara, T., Pal, B., Ferdous, Z., Esha, S. N., Patwary, H., & Rahman, M. M. (2025). Prevalence and correlates of anxiety and depression among ever-married reproductive-aged women in Bangladesh: National-level insights from the 2022 Bangladesh Demographic and Health Survey. *BMC Public Health, 25*(1), 1143.

Costello, E. J., Pine, D. S., Hammen, C., March, J. S., Plotsky, P. M., Weissman, M. M., Biederman, J., Goldsmith, H. H., Kaufman, J., Lewinsohn, P. M., & Hellander, M. (2002). Development and natural history of mood disorders. *Biological psychiatry, 52*(6), 529–542.

Prakash, P. (2022). *Textbook of mental health & psychiatric nursing for BSc students: As per the syllabus of Indian Nursing Council*. CBS Publishers & Distributors Pvt Ltd.

Sreevani, R. (2020). *A textbook of mental health (psychiatric) nursing* (4th ed.). Jaypee Brothers Medical Publishers.

Martin-Key, N. A., Olmert, T., Barton-Owen, G., Han, S. Y. S., Cooper, J. D., Eljasz, P., Farrag, L. P., Friend, L. V., Bell, E., Cowell, D., & Tomasik, J. (2021). The delta study-prevalence and characteristics of mood disorders in 924 individuals with low mood: Results of the of the World Health Organization Composite International Diagnostic Interview (CIDI). *Brain and Behavior, 11*(6), Article e02167.

Kalin, N. H. (2020). Advances in understanding and treating mood disorders. *American Journal of Psychiatry, 177*(8), 647–650.

Lee, H. J., Kim, S. H., & Lee, M. S. (2019). Understanding mood disorders in children. In *Frontiers in psychiatry: Artificial intelligence, precision medicine, and other paradigm shifts* (pp. 251–261). Springer Singapore.

Chapter 7
Care of Clients with Anxiety Disorders

Ravi Philip Rajkumar and S. M. Yasir Arafat

Abstract Anxiety disorders are among the most common mental disorders, affecting 5% of the world's population. These disorders are characterized by excessive or inappropriate levels of anxiety and anxiety-related symptoms, causing difficulties in carrying out normal activities. There are several types of anxiety disorders—generalized anxiety disorder, panic disorder, social anxiety disorder, specific phobia, and agoraphobia. These are distinguished based on the presence or absence of specific triggers and on their symptom profile. If untreated, anxiety disorders can cause significant impairment in interpersonal and social relationships, education, and employment. Anxiety disorders can be treated with medications, psychological interventions, or a combination of both. Nurses play an active role in the care of anxiety disorders in community and clinic settings. This chapter provides an overview of the symptoms, diagnosis, and treatment of anxiety disorders, and outlines the role of nurses in evaluating and managing patients who present with these conditions.

Keywords Anxiety disorders · Nursing care · Bangladesh · BSc Nursing · Psychiatric Nursing

1 Definitions and Concepts

Anxiety is a normal emotion that all of us experience as part of day-to-day life. It can be defined as an unpleasant or "uneasy" state, characterized by apprehension about an actual or imagined threat (Box 1). Anxiety is similar to fear, but fear involves the response to an actual danger, while anxiety occurs in **expectation** of danger. For

R. P. Rajkumar
Department of Psychiatry, Jawaharlal Institute of Postgraduate Medical Education and Research (JIPMER), puducherry, India
e-mail: ravi.psych@gmail.com

S. M. Y. Arafat (✉)
Department of Psychiatry, Bangladesh Specialized Hospital, Dhaka, Bangladesh
e-mail: arafatdmc62@gmail.com

S. M. Y. Arafat and H. Akter (eds.), *Psychiatric Nursing in Bangladesh*, Mental Health Systems and Policy in Low- and Middle-Income Countries,
https://doi.org/10.1007/978-981-95-8501-4_7

example, if a person sees a poisonous snake, he will experience fear. If he has been told that poisonous snakes have been spotted on a particular road, he will experience anxiety when walking there, even if he does not actually see a snake. Anxiety is often accompanied by physical changes such as increased perspiration, a faster heart rate, and rapid breathing.

Real or potential threats are also known as **"stressors"** or "stressful events." In daily life, stressors are commonly encountered in the setting of academics, work, relationships, family, and finances. A "normal" level of anxiety is part of the natural **"stress response,"** which helps us to focus on specific problems or challenges. For example, anxiety before an examination can motivate a student to set aside distractions and spend more time studying. However, some people experience excessive levels of anxiety, which are either out of proportion to the stressor, or occur even in the absence of a stressor. Such abnormally high levels of anxiety are associated with other physical or psychological symptoms, and interfere with the person's ability to function normally. Patients with these problems are said to have **anxiety disorders**.

Anxiety disorders can be broadly divided into **phobias** and other anxiety disorders. The word "phobia" comes from the Greek *phobos*, meaning "fear." A phobia is an anxiety disorder characterized by anxiety confined to, and triggered by, specific objects or situations. Other anxiety disorders are characterized by excessive anxiety that is not clearly related to a particular trigger or situation.

Box 1: Terms and definitions

Anxiety: A negative (unpleasant) emotion occurring in anticipation of a real or imagined threat or challenge.
Stressor: A challenging or threatening event experienced in the course of one's life.
Stress response: A natural response to a challenge or threat, involving physical and mental changes that prepare a person to handle the challenging situation.
Anxiety disorders: Mental illnesses or disorders characterized by excessive or abnormal anxiety.
Phobia: A mental disorder in which excessive anxiety occurs only in response to specific objects or situations.

2 Classification

Healthcare workers use two main systems to classify and diagnose anxiety disorders. The first is the *World Health Organization's International Classification of Diseases*, which is currently in its eleventh version **(ICD-11)**. The second is the American Psychiatric Association's Diagnostic and Statistical Manual of Mental Disorders, which is in its fifth edition **(DSM-5)**. Both systems use the same categories and nomenclature, though some diagnostic criteria for each disorder differ slightly. The ICD-11 is the system most used in South Asian countries. Box 2 provides a list of the different types of anxiety disorder.

Box 2: Types of anxiety disorder recognized by ICD-11 and DSM-5

- Generalized anxiety disorder (GAD).
- Panic disorder (PD).
- Agoraphobia.
- Specific phobia (also called simple phobia) (SP).
- Social anxiety disorder (also called social phobia) (SAD).
- Separation anxiety disorder.
- Selective mutism.
- Other specified anxiety disorder.
- Anxiety disorder, unspecified.

Among these conditions, separation anxiety disorder and selective mutism are usually seen only in children and adolescents. The terms "other specified anxiety disorder" and "anxiety disorder, unspecified" are used when patients have symptoms suggesting an anxiety disorder, but do not fit clearly into any of the defined types.

In some persons, symptoms of anxiety may be caused by a medical or neurological illness, or by the effects of drugs of abuse. For example:

- Persons with over-activity of the thyroid gland (**hyperthyroidism**) can experience symptoms of anxiety, irritability, palpitations, and increased sweating, resembling those of GAD.
- Persons with epilepsy arising from the temporal lobe of the brain may experience brief, intense episodes of anxiety which resemble panic attacks.
- Persons with alcohol withdrawal can experience symptoms of anxiety, restlessness, irritability, increased sweating, and rapid breathing. These resemble GAD or PD, but subside after 3–7 days of appropriate treatment.

In the first two cases, the patient would receive a diagnosis of **"secondary anxiety syndrome"** in ICD-11 and **"anxiety disorder due to another medical condition"** in DSM-5. In the third, the diagnosis in both systems would be **"substance-induced anxiety disorder"** related to alcohol.

3 Signs and Symptoms

The classification of anxiety disorders is based on specific signs and symptoms. These are described in Box 3. To diagnose a given anxiety disorder, the relevant symptoms should be present for **two or more months**. The symptoms should not occur only as part of another mental illness, such as depression. They should not be caused by a medical or neurological illness, or by the effects of a drug of abuse, as discussed above.

Box 3: Symptoms of individual anxiety disorders

Generalized anxiety disorder

- **"Free-floating" anxiety** which is not limited to any one situation or object.
- **Excessive worry** about negative events related to daily life.
- Associated physical symptoms of **muscle tension**, dry mouth, nausea, abdominal discomfort, palpitations, and tremors.
- Associated irritability, difficulty in concentration, and difficulty in falling or staying asleep.

Panic disorder

- Recurrent episodes of severe anxiety or fear, known as **panic attacks**, lasting anywhere from 5 to 60 minutes. (see box 5).
- Episodes usually occur without a trigger, or "out of the blue," and rapidly reach a "peak" before subsiding.
- Between episodes, patients worry about having future episodes (**anticipatory anxiety**).

Over time, attacks may recur in association with the place or situation, but the person is not afraid of that place or situation.

Agoraphobia

- Abnormal anxiety associated with situations from which escape is considered difficult, or where help is not available. E.g., crowds, public transport, open spaces, or large buildings.
- Exposure to the feared situation often triggers a panic attack.
- Patients worry that they will either have a panic attack or "embarrassing" symptoms (such as vomiting, fainting, or incontinence) if exposed to the situation again.

Patients actively avoid the places or situations that trigger this fear.

Specific phobia

- Abnormal anxiety associated with exposure to a specific object or situation.
- Common triggers for phobias include domestic animals (e.g., dogs or cats), insects, heights, air travel, the sight of blood, or receiving injections.
- Patients sometimes report more than one specific trigger for their fear.

Patients actively avoid the object or situation involved and experience severe anxiety or fear if they cannot do so.

Social anxiety disorder

- Abnormal anxiety triggered by social situations (e.g., taking to a new person, eating in public) or performance situations (e.g., delivering a speech, answering a question in a classroom).
- Fear of being scrutinized, criticized, or mocked by others.
- The patient worries about either behaving inappropriately (e.g., forgetting an answer) or experiencing symptoms of anxiety in these situations, leading to fear of embarrassment or humiliation.

Patients either avoid social / performance situations or experience severe anxiety when exposed to them.

Panic attacks can be seen both in PD and in other anxiety disorders. The identification of a panic attack is important in hospital settings, as it is often misdiagnosed as a cardiac or respiratory problem (Box 4).

Box 4: Symptoms of a panic attack

- Breathing difficulties—Shortness of breath; "choking sensations".
- Cardiovascular symptoms—Chest pain or discomfort; palpitations.
- Gastrointestinal symptoms—Abdominal discomfort; nausea.
- Neurological symptoms—Dizziness; feelings of cold or heat; tremors; increased perspiration.
- Psychological symptoms—Feelings of unreality of the self (**depersonalization**) or of the environment (**derealization**); fears of dying, going "mad," or "losing control".

To diagnose a panic attack, several (at least **four**) of these symptoms should be present, and should rapidly worsen before gradually settling. Recurrent episodes with three or fewer symptoms are present, or without a typical "peak," are known as **partial symptom panic attacks**.

4 The Concept of Anxiety in Nursing

The DSM-5 and ICD-11 criteria are used by mental health professionals when diagnosing and treating persons with anxiety disorders. Hildegard Peplau, often considered the "mother of psychiatric nursing," outlined a different approach to classifying symptoms of anxiety. Peplau's system is not meant for diagnostic purposes, but to help nurses to "grade" the severity of a person's anxiety and to provide appropriate nursing interventions. This system is described in Table 1.

NANDA International (NANDA-I), a global nurses' association focused on standardizing nursing terminology, has included anxiety in its list of nursing diagnoses. The NANDA-I definition of anxiety is "a vague, uneasy feeling of discomfort or dread accompanied by an autonomic response; a feeling of apprehension caused by anticipation of danger. It is an alerting sign that warns of impending danger and enables the individual to take measures to deal with the threat." NANDA-I guidelines recommend that patients experiencing anxiety should undergo further evaluation by the nurse in charge. This will help them decide whether they are suffering from an anxiety disorder and in need of treatment.

Table 1 Peplau's levels of anxiety

Level	Description	Significance
Mild	A mild feeling of anxiety or apprehension. Symptoms of restlessness, irritability, and behaviours such as nail-biting or fidgeting.	Normal. Can help a person to focus on a specific problem or situation.
Moderate	Activation of the stress response, with reduced attention to the environment. Symptoms of increased perspiration, headache, gastric discomfort, and tremors.	May indicate an anxiety disorder or a response to a significant stressor.
Severe	Marked anxiety and distress, and full activation of the stress response. Difficulty in concentrating, remembering, or solving problems. Symptoms as in moderate anxiety, along with rapid breathing, disturbed sleep, and a sense that "something bad" will happen soon.	Indicates the presence of an anxiety disorder or anxiety symptoms as part of another mental disorder. Can also occur in response to a severe or traumatic stressor.
Panic	Extreme levels of anxiety, with marked agitation and restlessness or marked withdrawal. Symptoms as in the above, but may sometimes include illusions or hallucinations.	Can be seen during panic attacks, during acute exacerbations of an anxiety disorder, or in relation to substance abuse (e.g., during alcohol withdrawal). May also indicate a severe mental illness or delirium (see the relevant chapters).

Epidemiology

At least 4% of the world's population, or approximately 300 million people, suffer from an anxiety disorder. The prevalence of these disorders is higher (about 7–8%) in North and South America. In South Asian countries, anxiety is estimated to affect 3–5% of the general population. Phobic disorders (SP and SAD) are more common than other anxiety disorders (GAD, PD, and agoraphobia), with an approximate ratio of 3:2.

Anxiety disorders are approximately 1.5 to 2 times more common in women than in men. The age at onset of anxiety disorders varies across individual types. SAD and SP commonly begin in late childhood or early adolescence. GAD, PD, and agoraphobia have a later onset, and usually appear at 20–35 years of age.

Risk Factors for Anxiety Disorders

Anxiety disorders result from an interaction between genes and the environment. About 30–40% of the risk for these disorders is genetic. This risk arises from multiple genetic variants and cannot be attributed to a single gene or mutation. First-degree relatives of persons with an anxiety disorder—that is, parents and siblings—are 4 to 6 times more likely to develop an anxiety disorder.

Adverse experiences during childhood, such as the loss of a parent, childhood abuse or neglect, or witnessing domestic violence, increase the risk of anxiety disorders. Such experiences create a sense of insecurity in the growing child and an exaggerated perception of threat or danger. Because of this, even "normal" stressors in later life can trigger the onset of an anxiety disorder in adults who have experienced childhood adversity.

Several other risk and protective factors have been identified by researchers. These are summarized in Table 2.

Because these factors are modifiable, they are amenable to public health interventions. Positive coping and attribution styles can be taught as part of life skills education in schools and colleges. Health promotion activities and lifestyle interventions at the community level can promote physical exercise and the avoidance of substances of abuse. Workplace mental health services can be developed to strengthen social support, improve communication between members of an organization, and

Table 2 Modifiable risk and protective factors for anxiety disorders

Factor	Significance
Tobacco use	• Cigarette smoking associated with agoraphobia and PD • Smoking frequency increases risk of all anxiety disorders
Alcohol use	• Higher consumption of alcohol is associated with anxiety disorders in women, but not in men
Cannabis use	• Cannabis use in adolescents is associated with an elevated risk of SAD
Appraisal style	• A tendency to interpret daily events in a negative or threatening manner may increase the risk of anxiety disorders in general
Coping style	• "Avoidant" coping, in which a person tries to avoid or delay facing problems, increases the risk for anxiety disorders • Addressing stressors directly ("problem-focused coping"), or dealing effectively with negative emotions ("emotion-focused coping"), reduces the risk of specific phobia in women
Workplace factors	• High demands at work, conflicts with peers or superiors, and reduced job security increase the risk of GAD • Social support at work reduces the risk of GAD
Social support	• Low social support is associated with a higher risk of SAD
Physical activity	• Regular physical activity or exercise is associated with a lower risk of PD and agoraphobia

teach stress management or relaxation techniques. In this way, it may be possible to prevent anxiety disorders in the general population, or at least reduce their severity.

Symptoms of Anxiety in Other Psychiatric Disorders

Almost any psychiatric disorder may present with symptoms of anxiety. It is important to obtain a complete history and to consult all available records to ensure that the correct diagnosis is made. Conditions that are often confused with anxiety disorders are mentioned as depression, adjustment disorder, obsessive-compulsive disorder (OCD), post-traumatic stress disorder (PTSD), substance use disorders, schizophrenia, hypochondriasis, body dysmorphic disorder, and neurodevelopmental disorders. In most cases, the anxiety experienced by these patients responds to appropriate treatment of the underlying diagnosis, along with patient and caregiver education, and environmental modification if required.

Comorbidity between Anxiety Disorders and Other Mental Disorders

Patients with anxiety disorders may also suffer from other mental illnesses. This phenomenon is known as **comorbidity**. The patient often needs concurrent treatment of both conditions. The most common comorbid diagnosis in anxiety disorders is depression. It is estimated that persons with anxiety disorders are six times more likely to develop depression, and vice versa. Approximate rates of comorbidity between other psychiatric disorders and anxiety disorders are given in Table 3.

Nurses working in general hospital or primary care settings should be aware that the distinction between depression, anxiety disorders, and bodily distress disorders is not always easy to make. Many patients present with a combination of depressive, anxious, and bodily symptoms which do not fit neatly into any category. In some cases, patients may fulfil criteria for more than one diagnosis (Table 3). In other

Table 3 Comorbidity in anxiety disorders

Disorder	Prevalence of anxiety disorders in persons with the disorder	Prevalence of the disorder in persons with anxiety disorders
Depression	30–50%	30–50%
Bipolar disorder	30–45%	5–15%
Substance use disorders	20–50%	20–45%
PTSD	35–40%	5–10%
OCD	25–50%	5–10%
Bodily distress disorders	10–45%	5–50%

cases, it may be more productive to focus on all existing symptoms rather than on a specific diagnosis, and to tailor treatment to each type of symptom—for example, to combine medications for depression with behavioural techniques for anxiety or bodily distress.

Cultural Factors in Anxiety Disorders

Cultural beliefs, values, and practices can affect anxiety disorders in at least three ways.

- Cultures vary in terms of the amount of support available from families and communities. Higher levels of social support may be protective against anxiety disorder, or help patients with an anxiety disorder to recover. Cultures that place a higher emphasis on individual achievements and competition may worsen anxiety disorders.
- Cultural attitudes may influence a patient's willingness to seek treatment from mental health professionals. In some cultures, mental illness may be seen as a punishment from God, or as caused by "black magic" or spirits. Persons with an anxiety disorder may experience discrimination due to such beliefs: this is known as **stigmatization**, and may make them less likely to receive proper treatment. Patients or caregivers who endorse these beliefs may choose magico-religious or traditional healing practices over mental health care.
- The symptoms of anxiety disorders vary across cultures. For example, patients in Asian countries may emphasize the physical symptoms of anxiety, such as dizziness or gastrointestinal discomfort, when consulting doctors. Sometimes, patients may report anxiety directly related to cultural beliefs. For example, male patients in India or Sri Lanka can present with anxiety related to "semen loss" through nocturnal emissions, known as **dhat syndrome**. Similarly, patients in South and Central America may present with panic attacks in the context of interpersonal problems, often associated with anger. They describe this as **ataque de nervios** ("nerve attack" in Spanish).

Course of Anxiety Disorders

If not treated, anxiety disorders tend to persist and run a chronic course. If appropriate treatment is provided, at least 60–70% of patients experience significant improvement. Trials of medication have shown sustained benefit for at least 1–2 years. Patients receiving psychological therapies have also been found to maintain improvement for over a year.

Studies that have followed up patients for 7 to 14 years have found that about 60% of patients with PD, 50% of patients with GAD, and 35–45% of patients with SAD or agoraphobia have good outcomes. The longest such study followed up patients with GAD for forty years. 83% of patients were seen to improve in the long run, and their symptoms tended to lessen or disappear after the age of 50. However, many of these patients continued to experience bodily distress symptoms later in life. In general, patients whose anxiety disorder begins at a younger age, or who do not follow prescribed treatments, have a worse outcome.

Patients with anxiety disorders experience difficulties in many aspects of their life if their symptoms are untreated. These include both psychosocial and medical complications, and are summarized in Box 5. Appropriate pharmacological and psychological treatment can prevent or resolve many of these adverse outcomes.

Box 5 Complications of untreated or persistent anxiety disorders

- Academic difficulties.
- Unemployment or impaired work performance.
- Marital disharmony and separation.
- Difficulties in social interaction.
- Substance use—As a form of "self-medication".
- Depression.
- Medical illnesses—Gastrointestinal, cardiovascular, musculoskeletal, and neurological.
- Memory impairment in late life.
- Suicide—Approximately four-fold increase in risk.

For nurses working in general hospital settings, it is important to note that anxiety disorders are associated with a wide range of medical illnesses. This link is **bidirectional**—patients with chronic medical illnesses can develop anxiety disorders due to the chronic stress associated with their physical condition, but patients with anxiety disorders are also more likely to develop some types of medical illness.

Assessment of a Patient with a Suspected Anxiety Disorder

Based on what we have learned so far, let us consider two case vignettes and understand how to evaluate patients with suspected anxiety disorders (Box 6).

Box 6: Clinical cases

Mr. C, a young man aged 25, presents to the emergency department of a general hospital with the complaint that "he thinks he is having a heart attack." On evaluation, he reports symptoms of palpitations, breathlessness, chest discomfort, and dizziness for the past 30 minutes, of sudden onset. Over the last four months, he has experienced ten episodes of this sort, and all of them last about 30 minutes to 1 hour. Each time he has an episode, he thinks that he might die. Between them, he often worries as to when he will get his next episode of "heart trouble." He is otherwise physically healthy and denies using alcohol, tobacco, or drugs of abuse. There is no family history of cardiac disease. On examination, his pulse rate is 102/min, his blood pressure is 120/82 mmHg, and his respiratory rate is 22/min. No abnormalities are identified on examining the cardiovascular and respiratory systems. Oxygen saturation on room air is 100%, his electrocardiogram (ECG) is normal, and his blood investigations, including serum troponin I, are normal. As the nursing staff in charge of this case, what do you think this patient is suffering from, and how can you help him in the setting of the emergency room?	Ms. D is a woman aged 30, working as a college lecturer. She has come to the psychiatry out-patient department with complaints of disturbed sleep and increased "tension" for the past eight months. On clarification of the history, it appears that these problems started when she was assigned additional teaching and administrative responsibilities by her principal, and found them difficult to manage. Since then, she frequently wakes up from sleep, experiences nightmares of losing her job or her children falling ill, and finds it hard to fall asleep thereafter. She spends several hours during the day worrying about various daily situations—her workload, her children's performance at school, and interpersonal conflicts with her sister-in-law. Her husband, who accompanies her, says that she often seems "impatient" and gets "irritated" easily. She finds it difficult to concentrate on the task at hand, and experiences headache and neck pain intermittently. On days when the college is closed, she is unable to feel "restful" even if she goes on an outing with her family. She does not report any feelings of sadness, negative thoughts about herself or the future, or any wishes to end her life. Her physical examination is unremarkable. During the psychiatric interview, she appears anxious and slightly restless. She reports repeated, frequent worries about her work and family. None of these worries appear unrealistic or bizarre: they are exaggerations of genuine concerns in her life. She is aware that her worrying is excessive, and says that she has come to seek help so that "she doesn't get tensed up so much." What is Ms. D's likely diagnosis, and what nursing interventions are effective for this kind of problem?

First, a careful history should be taken, and a proper physical examination should be carried out (Box 7).

Box 7: History-taking and physical examination in patients with anxiety disorders

History	Physical examination
• Symptoms of anxiety (Table 1) • Panic attacks (Box 3) • Duration of symptoms • Presence of stressful life events • Specific triggers for symptoms • Fear of specific objects or situations • Level of impairment or disability • Beliefs and attitudes regarding the symptoms • Symptoms of depression • Suicidal ideas or attempts • Substance use • Medical illnesses and treatment(s) taken for them • Current living arrangements and social support • Family history of similar complaints	• Body weight and body mass index (BMI) • Thyroid gland • Pulse rate and regularity • Blood pressure • Respiratory system—any abnormal breath sounds • Cardiovascular system—any murmurs or added sounds • Signs related to substance use—e.g., signs of liver involvement in patients with alcohol abuse • Scars or marks of self-injury or suicide attempts

Certain laboratory tests can also be useful in ruling out medical conditions that "mimic" anxiety disorders (Table 4). These tests need not be done routinely: they are indicated only if the history and examination suggest a medical cause. Nurses in charge of patients with symptoms of anxiety should ensure that they are carried out.

Table 4 Laboratory tests in patients with suspected anxiety disorders

Investigation	Significance
Thyroid function tests—Thyroid-stimulating hormone (TSH), free thyroxine (fT_4) tri-iodothyronine (fT_3)	To rule out hyperthyroidism, which can mimic either generalized anxiety disorder or panic disorder
Random blood glucose	To rule out hypoglycaemia (low blood sugar), which can mimic a panic attack
Liver function tests—Serum bilirubin, serum transaminases and gamma-glutamyl transferase	To rule out alcohol abuse and some forms of liver disease. Alcohol withdrawal can cause symptoms of anxiety. Chronic liver disease can lead to anxiety or panic attacks
Electrocardiogram (ECG)	To identify heart rhythm disturbances or ischemic heart disease. Both these conditions can mimic panic attacks
Electroencephalogram (EEG)	To rule out certain forms of epilepsy that can cause sudden fear or panic
Urine drug screening	To check for recent use or abuse substances such as cannabis, opioids, or benzodiazepines

The patient in **Case Vignette 1** probably suffers from panic disorder. He has experienced recurrent panic attacks with anticipatory anxiety and has no symptoms of generalized or phobic anxiety. His physical examination and laboratory investigations do not suggest any medical, neurological, or substance-related cause for his symptoms.

The patient in **Case Vignette 2** appears to have generalized anxiety disorder. She has "free-floating" worries related to several aspects of her everyday life, with no single situation or trigger, and no panic attacks. Her other symptoms, such as irritability and difficulty in relaxing, are also common in GAD.

Screening for Anxiety Disorders

Imagine that you are a psychiatric nurse involved in research at a general hospital. The aim of the project is to check whether patients seeking consultations for medical problems, such as body pain or cough, also have symptoms of anxiety. There may not be enough time to carry out a full assessment of each patient, and patients who are ill may not be able to cooperate with it. Specific short questionnaires, known as **screening instruments**, have been developed for use in these situations. A screening instrument consists of a limited number of questions, which are meant to identify common symptoms of anxiety. If a person scores above a certain "cut-off" on this instrument, it means that they have significant anxiety and need a detailed evaluation. Screening instruments are not meant to diagnose any specific anxiety disorder. Examples of commonly used screening instruments for anxiety are the Generalized Anxiety Disorder Scale-7 (GAD-7), the Hospital Anxiety and Depression Scale (HADS), and the Depression, Anxiety and Stress Scale (DASS-21). The GAD-7 is used to screen for anxiety alone, while the HADS and DASS-21 screen for both anxiety and depression.

Treatment for Anxiety Disorders

There are two main types of treatment for anxiety disorders: **pharmacotherapy** (medications) and **psychological interventions**. Often, the best outcomes are achieved by **combined** treatments, in which the most suitable medications and psychological interventions are selected based on the patient's clinical profile.

(a) **Pharmacotherapy for Anxiety Disorders.**

Several medications are available for the treatment of anxiety disorders. None of these completely "cure" the disorder. Instead, they bring about a substantial improvement in symptoms in many patients. This allows them to carry out their daily activities with little or no interference. Most medicines have a delayed onset of action, and should be taken for 4 to 8 weeks to determine their effectiveness. About 50–70% of patients respond well to medications.

Response to treatment with these drugs is usually through **rating scales** which measure symptoms of anxiety. Two commonly used rating scales are the *Hamilton Anxiety Rating Scale* for GAD and the *Liebowitz Social Anxiety Scale* for social anxiety disorder. Another measure that is often used is the Clinical Global Impression, which uses the assessing doctor or nurse's overall view of the patient's symptom severity and improvement.

Currently approved medications for anxiety disorders are described in Table 5.

Table 5 Medications used in the treatment of anxiety disorders

Drug	Starting dose	Maximum dose	Indications
A. Selective serotonin reuptake inhibitors (SSRIs) These drugs are generally considered the first line of treatment for anxiety disorders			
Escitalopram	5 mg/day	15–20 mg/day	GAD, PD, AP, SAD
Fluoxetine	20 mg/day	40–60 mg/day	PD, AP, GAD
Paroxetine	20 mg/day (plain) 12.5 mg/day (extended release)	40–60 mg/day (plain) 50–75 mg/day (extended release)	GAD, PD, SAD
Sertraline	25 mg/day	100–150 mg/day	GAD, PD, AP, SAD
B. Serotonin and noradrenaline reuptake inhibitors (SNRIs) These drugs are generally used when patients do not respond to SSRIs			
Venlafaxine	37.5 mg/day (extended release)	75–225 mg/day (extended release)	GAD, PD, SAD
Duloxetine	20–30 mg/day	60 mg/day	GAD
C. Benzodiazepines (BZDs) These drugs are used for short-term (1–2 months) relief of anxiety, and for insomnia associated with anxiety, or on an "as-needed" basis for acute anxiety			
Alprazolam	0.25–0.5 mg/day	1–4 mg/day	GAD, PD, AP
Clonazepam	0.5 mg/day	1–2 mg/day	PD, AP
Lorazepam	1–2 mg/day	4–6 mg/day	GAD, PD, insomnia due to anxiety
Oxazepam	15 mg/day	30–60 mg/day	Acute anxiety
D. Other drugs These drugs are generally used as "add-ons" in patients who respond partially to SSRIs or SNRIs. Propranolol can also be used on an "as-needed" basis			
Pregabalin	50–75 mg/day	300–600 mg/day	GAD, SAD
Propranolol	10–20 mg/day	40–120 mg/day	Situation-specific SAD, physical symptoms in GAD
Hydroxyzine	10 mg/day	25–50 mg/day	GAD

Abbreviations AP, agoraphobia; GAD, generalized anxiety disorder; PD, panic disorder; SAD, social anxiety disorder

Special caution is required with **benzodiazepines**, because patients taking them for three or more months may become dependent on them. Benzodiazepine dependence is similar in nature to alcohol dependence: persons experience a feeling of relaxation or a "high" when taking the drug, and experience anxiety, palpitations, insomnia, and irritability if it is suddenly discontinued. These are known as **withdrawal symptoms**. In severe cases, benzodiazepine withdrawal can lead to confusion or to seizures. The prescription of these drugs should be monitored carefully by the treating doctor or nurse. They should be gradually **tapered**—by reducing 25% of the dose every week over 4 weeks—after two months of use, to prevent abuse or dependence. Patients taking benzodiazepines should avoid driving or operating heavy machinery, because these drugs can increase the risk of an accident.

When using these drugs in patients above the age of 60, both the starting dose and the maximum dose should be half the doses mentioned in Table 6. Elderly patients are at a higher risk of hyponatremia and gastrointestinal haemorrhage when taking SSRIs or SNRIs. Benzodiazepines should be used cautiously in this age group, because of the risk of confusion, memory impairment, and falls.

When using SSRIs in adolescents or young adults (age < 25 years), patients should be monitored by the treating doctor or nurse every week for the first four weeks. This

Table 6 Summarizes the main psychological interventions for anxiety disorders

Intervention	Description	Indications
Cognitive-behavioural therapies (CBTs)	A combination of: (a) **cognitive** techniques to challenge mistaken thoughts or interpretations of stimuli (b) **Behavioural** techniques involving gradual confrontation of the feared stimulus, as in exposure therapy	GAD, SP, SAD, PD, AP
Exposure therapies	Step-wise exposure to feared stimuli or situations. Can be done through imagining the stimulus (**imaginal exposure**), actual exposure to the stimulus with the help of a therapist (**graded exposure**) or exposure to bodily sensations associated with panic attacks (**interoceptive exposure**)	SP (graded or imaginal exposure), SAD, PD (interoceptive exposure), AP. Can also be used for specific worries or concerns in GAD
Relaxation techniques	Includes deep breathing, progressive muscle relaxation, guided imagery, and other methods to activate the natural "relaxation response"	GAD; adjunctive role in other anxiety disorders
Mindfulness techniques	Involves focusing on the present moment and experiences, both internal and internal, from a "non-judgmental" perspective	GAD; adjunctive role in other anxiety disorders. Usually combined with CBT techniques

Abbreviations AP, agoraphobia; GAD, generalized anxiety disorder; PD, panic disorder; SAD, social anxiety disorder; SP, specific phobia

is because persons in this age group can experience rare but serious **behavioural changes**, including agitation, worsening of anxiety, and suicidal ideation, at the beginning of treatment. If such changes occur, the medication may need to be stopped or changed. Venlafaxine and paroxetine are not approved for use in patients below the age of 18 years.

These medications should be used with caution during pregnancy, especially during the first trimester, as their effect on the developing child is unknown. **Paroxetine** should be avoided during pregnancy, as it has been found to cause cardiac septal defects in infants. Newborn babies born to mothers taking SSRIs may experience a short-lasting "discontinuation syndrome," characterized by irritability, feeding difficulties, excessive crying, and/or disturbed sleep lasting one to two weeks. This syndrome is more common in pre-term infants.

SSRIs are the initial drugs of choice for all anxiety disorders, except specific phobia, for which no specific pharmacotherapy is available. Escitalopram and sertraline are preferred due to their tolerability and lack of interactions with other drugs. These should be started at the doses given in Table 7.5 and increased every 3–7 days until the maximum tolerated dose is reached. Patients should be educated about the time necessary for these medicines to start working: they will experience improvement only after two to four weeks of treatment. Once the "target" dose is reached, the medication should be continued for at least **6 to 8 weeks**, and the patient should be reviewed every 2 weeks to assess for a response. If a patient responds well to treatment, research suggests that the medication should be continued for at least **6 to 12 months.**

If a patient does not respond to an SSRI, either a second SSRI or an SNRI can be used. The previous medication should be tapered and stopped by reducing 25% of the dose every week, over a period of four weeks, and the new medication should be started in parallel with it. If the medication being stopped is fluoxetine, no tapering is necessary. The second medication should also be tried for 6 to 8 weeks at the maximum dose that the patient can tolerate. If there is a good response to treatment, it should be continued as described above.

Benzodiazepines are best used for the short-term treatment of acute anxiety, as "add-ons" during the first 2 to 4 weeks of SSRI or SNRI treatment. Once the patient starts responding to the SSRI or SNRI, BZDs should be tapered and stopped over a period of two to four weeks, reducing the dose by one-fourth every 3 to 7 days.

The other drugs mentioned in Table 5 are best prescribed by a psychiatrist with experience in the management of anxiety disorders.

The pharmacological management of anxiety disorders is summarized in Fig. 1.

b. Psychological Interventions

Psychological interventions or psychotherapies are an essential component of treatment for persons with anxiety disorders (Table 7.6). They can be used either by themselves, or in combination with medication. They are effective in patients who show only a partial response to medication, and in specific phobia, where there is no effective pharmacological treatment.

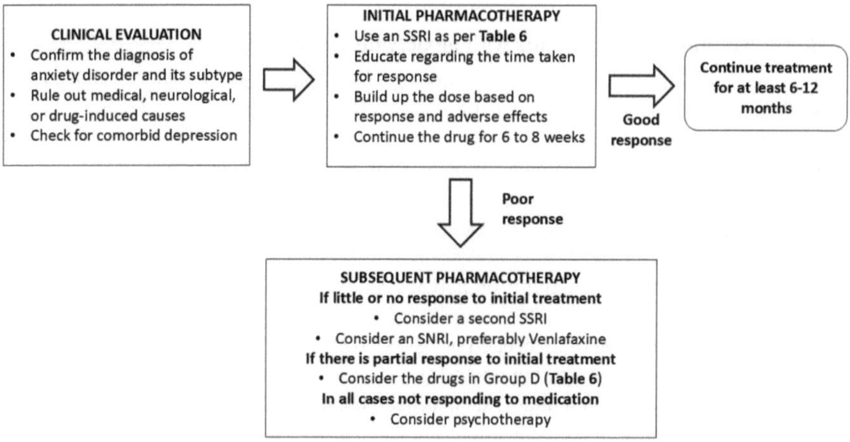

Fig. 1 Pharmacological management of anxiety disorders

CBT has the best supporting evidence for the treatment of anxiety disorders. Regardless of the specific method adopted, all psychological therapies should be preceded by patient education (**psychoeducation**), so that they understand the nature of their disorder and the way in which therapy works. Psychological interventions usually require 8 to 20 sessions to be effective; these sessions can be held once or twice a week, and the patient is given tasks (**"homework assignments"**) between sessions, to apply what they have learned from the therapist in "real life" settings. After the conclusion of therapy, patients may be seen once a month for two to three **"booster"** sessions to reinforce what they have learned about managing their anxiety. About 60–70% of patients with anxiety disorders respond well to psychological therapies. A major advantage of these therapies over medication is that their effect persists even after therapy sessions have stopped. Because of this, they are better than medication at preventing relapses of anxiety disorders.

There are no "side effects" of psychological therapies, though some patients may report an initial worsening of anxiety during exposure sessions. The major limitations of psychological therapies are that they require skilled therapists, who are not often available in low- and middle-income countries, as well as significant investments in terms of time, travel, and /or money on the part of the patient.

Nursing Interventions for Anxiety Disorders.

The nursing process can be beneficial for patients with anxiety disorders, even if nursing staff have not been formally trained in psychological therapies. Box 8 lists the fundamental components of nursing care when a patient is suspected of having an anxiety disorder. Research has shown that nurses can be very effective **care managers** of patients with these disorders, in collaboration with either a general physician or a psychiatrist.

Box 8: Nursing care of patients with anxiety disorders

- Assessment of the patient's level of anxiety (see Peplau's classification, Table 1).
- Educating the patient about the nature of their illness and the treatment being given to them (psychoeducation).
- Arranging a quiet environment for the patient, or shifting them to one.
- Allowing patients to express their concerns openly and listening to them.
- Reassurance regarding specific concerns (e.g., if a patient with PD thinks she is having a "heart attack").
- Encouraging physical activity or hobbies as distractions (for mild or moderate anxiety).
- Cautious prescription of as-needed or "SOS" BZDs (for severe anxiety or panic).
- Coordination with the treating doctor(s).
- Teaching relaxation techniques, such as deep breathing.
- Ensuring that prescribed medications are taken as advised.

The **Nursing Interventions Classification** (NIC) lists eight interventions that can be learned and applied by psychiatric nurses caring for patients with anxiety. These are: (1) anxiety reduction, (2) coping enhancement, (3) relaxation therapy, (4) counselling, (5) anger management, (6) crisis intervention, (7) relocation stress reduction, and (8) life story therapy. These techniques can be learned from an experienced psychiatric nurse-therapist.

Several nurse-led **complementary interventions** have been suggested for patients with anxiety disorders. These include yoga, music therapy, aromatherapy, and "therapeutic touch." Though their efficacy is not well established, they may be indicated on a case-by-case basis, particularly if patients are uncomfortable with conventional pharmacotherapy or psychotherapy.

Nursing Management of Anxiety Disorder

1. Assessment and Observation

- Assess Symptoms: Monitor for physical symptoms (e.g., tachycardia, sweating) and psychological symptoms (e.g., excessive worry, fear).
- Identify Triggers: Determine specific situations or factors exacerbating the patient's anxiety.
- Risk Assessment: Evaluate for suicidal ideation or self-harm risks.

2. Establish a Therapeutic Relationship

- Provide Emotional Support: Build trust by being empathetic, approachable, and non-judgmental.

- Ensure Safety: Create a calm and supportive environment to reduce anxiety triggers.
- Active Listening: Allow the patient to express feelings and fears openly.

3. Psychosocial Interventions

- **Teach Relaxation Techniques**:
- Deep breathing exercises.
- Progressive muscle relaxation.
- Mindfulness or grounding exercises.
- **Encourage Positive Coping Strategies**:
- Journaling or writing about emotions.
- Encouraging participation in therapeutic activities, such as art or music therapy.
- **Gradual Exposure**: Assist the patient in facing anxiety-inducing situations in a controlled, supportive manner.

4. Medication Administration and Monitoring

- Administer Prescribed Medications:
- Antidepressants (e.g., SSRIs like Sertraline).
- Anxiolytics (e.g., Benzodiazepines like Lorazepam for short-term use).
- Beta-blockers (e.g., Propranolol for physical symptoms).
- Monitor for Side Effects: Observe for adverse effects of medications, such as drowsiness or dependency on benzodiazepines.

5. Psychoeducation

- Patient Education: Teach about the nature of anxiety, treatment options, and the importance of adherence to therapy.
- Family Involvement: Educate family members to provide support and reduce stigma.

6. Environmental Modifications

- Minimize Stimuli: Reduce loud noises, bright lights, and chaotic situations in the ward.
- Provide a Safe Space: Offer a quiet room or area for relaxation when the patient feels overwhelmed.

7. Promote Healthy Lifestyle

- Encourage regular exercise, a balanced diet, and adequate sleep.
- Discourage caffeine, nicotine, and alcohol use.

8. Continuous Monitoring and Evaluation

- Regularly reassess the patient's progress and response to interventions.
- Modify the care plan as needed to address new challenges or symptoms.

5 Summary

Anxiety disorders are common both in the general population and in hospital settings. These conditions are characterized by excessive levels of anxiety, with associated mental or physical discomfort and impairment in daily activities. Patients presenting with symptoms of excessive anxiety should be evaluated for medical, neurological, or drug-related causes before diagnosing an anxiety disorder. Nurses, whether in general hospital, emergency, or psychiatric settings, play a pivotal role in the assessment and treatment of anxiety disorders. Nursing care for these patients involves a combination of general, supportive interventions and specific therapy techniques that can be learned from trained experts.

Take Home Points

- Anxiety disorders are common psychiatric disorder.
- At least 4% of the world's population, or approximately 300 million people, suffer from an anxiety disorder.
- In South Asian countries, anxiety is estimated to affect 3–5% of the general population.
- Anxiety disorders are approximately 1.5 to 2 times more common in women than in men.
- Psychological interventions or psychotherapies are an essential component of treatment for persons with anxiety disorders.
- The nursing process can be beneficial for patients with anxiety disorders, even if nursing staff have not been formally trained in psychological therapies.

Sample Short Answer Questions

1. Define anxiety disorders.
2. Write down the causes/etiology/risk factors of anxiety disorders.
3. Write down the signs and symptoms of anxiety disorders.
4. Write down the clinical features of panic disorders.
5. Mention some examples of specific phobias.
6. What do you mean by phobia?

Sample Essay Questions

1. Explain the types of anxiety disorders according to ICD-11.
2. Explain the medical management of anxiety disorder.
3. As a psychiatric nurse, how will you manage a case of anxiety disorder in your ward?
4. How will you manage a case of agoraphobia?

Sample Multiple Choice Questions (MCQ) and Sample Best Answer Question

Etiology of anxiety disorders involves			Which factor is known to contribute to anxiety disorders?		
T	a)	Genetic factors contribute		a)	Only lifestyle choices
F	b)	Only external events cause anxiety	✓	b)	Genetic predisposition
T	c)	Neurotransmitter imbalances play a role		c)	Lack of exercise
F	d)	Anxiety is not just psychological		d)	Only positive experiences
T	e)	Stressors can trigger anxiety			

Suggested Reading

Anne Fishel. "Nursing management of anxiety and panic." Nursing Clinics of North America, vol. 33, no. 1, pp. 135–151.

Deborah Antai-Ontong. "Caring for the patient with an anxiety disorder." Nursing Clinics of North America, vol. 51, no. 2, pp. 173–183.

Open Resources for Nursing (Open RN). (2022) Ernstmeyer K, Christman E, editors. Nursing: Mental health and community concepts [internet]. Eau Claire (WI): Chippewa Valley Technical College. Chapter 9: Anxiety Disorders. Available from: https://www.ncbi.nlm.nih.gov/books/NBK590031/

Chapter 8
Care of Clients with Psychosomatic Illnesses and Somatoform Disorders

Bithika Mali, Hasina Akter, and S. M. Yasir Arafat

Abstract Somatoform and psychosomatic disorders encompass a spectrum of conditions in which psychological factors play a prominent role in the onset, maintenance, or exaggeration of physical symptoms. This chapter reviews definitions, contemporary classification schemes, etiology and risk factors, clinical presentation, diagnostic criteria, and evidence-based medical and nursing management. Emphasis is placed on a biopsychosocial model, integrated care approaches, and practical nursing interventions that improve patient outcomes and reduce unnecessary healthcare utilization. Practical case-focused guidance and structured nursing care plans are provided to facilitate clinical transformation in both acute and community settings.

Keywords Somatoform disorders · Somatization · Psychosomatic · Somatic symptom disorder · Conversion disorder · Nursing interventions · Biopsychosocial model

The boundaries between mind and body are permeable. Somatoform and psychosomatic disorders show how psychological processes can manifest as physical symptoms, leading to substantial distress and functional impairment. These conditions are frequently encountered across primary care, specialty clinics, and inpatient settings. Clinicians often face diagnostic and therapeutic challenges: patients present with genuine physical complaints, but evaluations reveal no sufficient organic explanation for the symptoms. This chapter synthesizes contemporary nosology or medical specialty, pathophysiology, diagnostic frameworks, and pragmatic management strategies with particular attention to nursing roles.

B. Mali · H. Akter
Department of Graduate Nursing, Bangladesh Medical University, Dhaka, Bangladesh

S. M. Y. Arafat (✉)
Department of Psychiatry, Bangladesh Specialized Hospital, Dhaka, Bangladesh
e-mail: arafatdmc62@gmail.com

S. M. Y. Arafat and H. Akter (eds.), *Psychiatric Nursing in Bangladesh*, Mental Health Systems and Policy in Low- and Middle-Income Countries,
https://doi.org/10.1007/978-981-95-8501-4_8

1 Definitions

Psychosomatic Illnesses

Psychosomatic illnesses are conditions in which psychological factors (stress, emotions, and personality traits) significantly contribute to the onset, exacerbation, or maintenance of physical disease. Historically, the term has been used to describe disorders such as essential hypertension, peptic ulcer disease, bronchial asthma, and some functional gastrointestinal disorders where psychological stressors modulate pathophysiology.

Somatoform Disorders

Somatoform disorders refer to a group of psychiatric syndromes characterized by persistent physical symptoms that are not fully explained by a physiological and pathological explanations justifying the symptoms. The patient's experience of symptoms is real; these are not fabricated or intentionally produced. Additionally, there is a disproportionate degree of preoccupation manifested by thought, feeling, and behavior and disability associated with somatic complaints. Functional impairment is a significant criteria to look for.

Somatization

Somatization is the process by which psychological distress is expressed through bodily complaints/physical symptoms. It can be a trait-like tendency or a state associated with acute stress or psychiatric disorder. Somatization may confer secondary gains such as attention or removal from stressful obligations that reinforce symptom persistence.

Classification

Modern classification systems have sought to reframe somatoform conditions to emphasize symptom burden and maladaptive health-related behaviors rather than the absence of disease. Two principal taxonomies are used internationally: *International Classification of Diseases* (ICD-11) and *Diagnostic and Statistical Manual of Mental Disorders* (DSM-5).

ICD-11: Disorders with Somatic Symptoms and Related Disorders

ICD-11 groups these conditions under 'Disorders with Somatic Symptoms or Bodily Distress.'

Key diagnostic categories include:

- Bodily Distress Disorder (BDD): persistent somatic symptoms with excessive attention, concern, or preoccupation.
- Conversion Disorder (Functional Neurological Symptom Disorder): neurological symptoms incompatible with recognized neurological disease.
- Other specified or unspecified bodily distress and somatic symptom conditions.

ICD-11 emphasizes a dimensional approach focusing on symptom severity, degree of health-related preoccupation, and functional impact. Types commonly described are:

1. Bodily Distress Disorder (mild, moderate, severe)—classified by the number and intensity of symptoms and the degree of cognitive and behavioral responses.
2. Functional Neurological Symptom Disorder (Conversion Disorder)—neurological symptoms (e.g., weakness, sensory disturbance, non-epileptic seizures) inconsistent with recognized pathology.
3. Persistent pain disorder where pain predominates and is associated with excessive health anxiety and disability.
4. Other specified and unspecified somatic symptom disorders used when presentation does not meet full criteria for a named disorder.

DSM-5: Somatic Symptom and Related Disorders

DSM-5 reframed somatoform disorders into 'Somatic Symptom and Related Disorders' (SSRDs). Major categories include:

- Somatic Symptom Disorder (SSD): one or more somatic symptoms that are distressing and accompanied by excessive thoughts, feelings, or behaviors.
- Illness Anxiety Disorder: preoccupation with having or acquiring a serious illness with minimal somatic symptoms.
- Conversion Disorder (Functional Neurological Symptom Disorder).
- Factitious or Artificial Disorder and Psychological Factors Affecting Other Medical Conditions are included in the broader chapter.

Epidemiology

Somatic symptom presentations are common in primary care. Epidemiological facts vary by setting and definition; however, estimates suggest that a significant proportion of primary care visits involve predominantly unexplained physical symptoms. Multiple risk factors—biological, psychological, and social interact—to produce vulnerability (Box 1).

Biological and Neurobiological Factors

Evidence implicates genetic predisposition to anxiety and depressive disorders, altered central and peripheral nervous system processing of sensory input, and dysregulation of neuroendocrine systems (HPA axis). Functional neuroimaging studies have shown altered activity in brain regions involved in emotion and interoception (e.g., anterior insula, anterior cingulate cortex) in patients with functional somatic disorders.

Psychological Factors

Psychological vulnerabilities include alexithymia (difficulty identifying and describing emotions), catastrophic thinking, illness beliefs that emphasize seriousness and threat, maladaptive coping strategies (avoidance, hypervigilance), and history of trauma or adverse childhood experiences.

Social and Cultural Factors

Social determinants such as low socioeconomic status, limited access to care, and cultural norms that favor somatic expressions of distress increase risk. Family dynamics that reinforce sick role behavior and frequent medicalization of normal bodily sensations are important contributors.

Box 1: Epidemiology and Risk Factors

Epidemiology

- Somatic symptom presentations are **common in primary care**.
- A **significant proportion** of primary care visits involve **unexplained physical symptoms**.
- **Prevalence rates vary** depending on the **definition** and **clinical setting**.

Biological and Neurobiological Factors

- **Genetic predisposition** to anxiety and depressive disorders.
- **Altered sensory processing** in the central and peripheral nervous systems.
- **Neuroendocrine dysregulation** (e.g., **HPA axis** abnormalities).
- **Functional neuroimaging** shows altered activity in regions like the **anterior insula** and **anterior cingulate cortex**, linked to emotion and interoception.

Psychological Factors

- **Alexithymia** (difficulty identifying and expressing emotions).
- **Catastrophic thinking** and **negative illness beliefs** (seeing bodily symptoms as serious/threatening).
- **Maladaptive coping** (e.g., avoidance, hypervigilance).
- **History of trauma** or **adverse childhood experiences** increases vulnerability.

Social and Cultural Factors

- **Low socioeconomic status** and **limited healthcare access**.
- **Cultural norms** promoting **somatic expression of distress**.
- **Family dynamics** that reinforce **sick-role behavior**.
- **Frequent medicalization** of normal bodily sensations contributes to chronicity.

Clinical Presentation

Clinical features can be diverse and multisystemic. Common presentations include persistent pain syndromes, chronic fatigue, gastrointestinal complaints (e.g., irritable bowel symptoms), cardiorespiratory sensations (palpitations, dyspnea), neurologic like symptoms (paresthesia, weakness), and non-epileptic seizures.

Typical behavioral and psychological features accompanying somatic symptoms include:

- Excessive health anxiety and repeated medical consultations.
- Preoccupation with symptom meaning and -disastrous interpretations.
- High healthcare utilization with multiple investigations and specialist referrals.
- Functional impairment in occupational, social, and interpersonal domains.
- Co-occurring mood and anxiety disorders are common.

2 Signs/Symptoms of Somatoform Disorder

Physical Symptoms

1. **Multiple, Non-Specific Symptoms**
   - Persistent pain (e.g., headaches, back pain, abdominal pain).
   - Gastrointestinal complaints (e.g., nausea, bloating, diarrhea).
   - Neurological symptoms (e.g., dizziness, paralysis, fainting).
   - Cardiopulmonary symptoms (e.g., chest pain, palpitations, shortness of breath).
2. **Disproportionate Physical Concerns**
   - Minor bodily sensations are perceived as severe or life-threatening.

Psychological Symptoms

1. **Excessive Preoccupation with Symptoms**
   - Persistent worry about the seriousness of physical complaints.
   - Fear of having a severe undiagnosed illness (e.g., cancer, heart disease).
2. **High Health-Related Anxiety**
   - Frequent checking or monitoring of bodily sensations.
   - Seeking repeated medical evaluations despite negative results.
3. **Maladaptive Thought Patterns**
   - Catastrophic thinking about symptoms.
   - Belief that symptoms are not adequately addressed by healthcare providers.

Behavioral Symptoms

1. **Frequent Medical Visits**:
   - Visiting multiple doctors or specialists without satisfaction from medical advice or test results.
   - Undergoing unnecessary diagnostic tests or procedures.
2. **Avoidance Behaviors**:
   - Avoiding activities or situations out of fear of worsening symptoms.
3. **Excessive Focus on Health**:
   - Spending excessive time and energy on managing symptoms.
4. **Non-Compliance with Medical Advice**:
   - Ignoring reassurances or advice from healthcare providers.

Emotional Symptoms

1. **Frustration or Anger**:
    - Feeling misunderstood or dismissed by healthcare providers.
2. **Mood Disturbances**:
    - Co-occurring anxiety or depression due to persistent health concerns.

Social Symptoms

1. **Impact on Daily Functioning**:
    - Difficulty maintaining work, school, or social relationships due to preoccupation with symptoms.
2. **Dependency**:
    - Relying heavily on family or caregivers for emotional or physical support.

Diagnostic Evaluation and DSM-5 Criteria

Diagnosis is clinical and rests on a careful history, targeted physical examination, and judicious use of investigations to exclude specific organic pathology. Importantly, DSM-5 focuses on positive psychological features (excessive thoughts, feelings, and behaviors) rather than absence of disease.

1. **DSM-5 Diagnostic Criteria for Somatic Symptom Disorder (SSD)**

DSM-5, SSD is diagnosed when:

a. One or more somatic symptoms that are distressing or result in significant disruption of daily life.
b. Excessive thoughts, feelings, or behaviors related to the symptoms, manifested by at least one of the following: disproportionate and persistent thoughts about the seriousness of the symptoms; persistently high anxiety about health or symptoms; excessive time and energy devoted to these symptoms or health concerns.
c. Although any one somatic symptom may not be continuously present, the state of being symptomatic is persistent (typically more than 6 months).
d. DSM-5 also emphasizes ruling out symptoms intentionally produced (artificial disorder) or feigned (malingering) and considering cultural context.

2. **Illness Anxiety Disorder (Hypochondriasis)**

Characterized by preoccupation with having or acquiring a serious illness. Somatic symptoms are not prominent or are very mild; the central feature is health anxiety and persistent reassurance-seeking.

3. **Conversion Disorder (Functional Neurological Symptom Disorder)**

Presents with neurological symptoms (motor or sensory) that are incompatible with established neurological disease. Diagnosis often requires neurologic examination demonstrating internal inconsistency and may involve collaboration with neurology.

3 Conversion Disorder

Conversion Disorder, also known as Functional Neurological Symptom Disorder, is a mental health condition where a person experiences neurological symptoms (e.g., paralysis, blindness, seizures) that are inconsistent with known medical or neurological conditions and cannot be explained by physical illness (Box 2). These symptoms are thought to be a result of psychological stress or trauma (Box 3). The nursing management is mentioned in Box 4.

Box 2: Signs/Symptoms of Conversion Disorder

- Motor Symptoms: Paralysis, weakness, tremors, abnormal gait.
- Sensory Symptoms: Blindness, deafness, numbness.
- Speech Disturbances: Mutism, slurred speech.
- Seizure-like Episodes: Psychogenic non-epileptic seizures (PNES).
- Coordination Issues: Difficulty walking, balance problems.

Box 3: Risk Factors of Conversion Disorder

- Psychological Stress: Trauma, abuse, conflict, or extreme stress can trigger symptoms.
- Maladaptive Coping Mechanisms: The mind converts emotional distress into physical symptoms.
- Comorbid Mental Disorders: Often associated with depression, anxiety, or PTSD.
- Social and Cultural Influences: More common in cultures where expressing emotions openly is discouraged.
- Psychological Stress: Trauma, abuse, conflict, or extreme stress can trigger symptoms.
- Maladaptive Coping Mechanisms: The mind converts emotional distress into physical symptoms.

DSM-5 Criteria of Conversion Disorder

- Based on clinical evaluation, excluding medical causes.

- **DSM-5 Criteria**:
  - Symptoms affect voluntary motor or sensory function.
  - No medical explanation for symptoms.
  - Significant distress or impairment in daily life.

Treatment and Management

- **Psychotherapy (First-Line Treatment)**: Explorative psychotherapy, problem-solving psychotherapy, interpersonal psychotherapy
- **Physical Therapy:** Prevents complications from immobility.
- **Medication:** Used for comorbid anxiety or depression.
- **Supportive Counseling:** Encourages coping strategies.

Box 4: Nursing Management of Conversion Disorder

- Therapeutic Communication: Build trust, validate concerns.
- Assessment: Identify stressors and triggers.
- Encourage Expression: Promote verbalizing emotions instead of physical symptoms.
- Rehabilitation Support: Assist with physical therapy and daily activities.
- Patient and Family Education: Teach about the condition and coping strategies.

4 Personality Disorders

Personality Disorders (PDs) are a group of mental health conditions characterized by persistent patterns of thinking, feeling, and behaving that deviate from societal expectations. These patterns cause distress and impair social, occupational, or personal functioning. Clinical presentation is mentioned in Box 5; potential risk factors are mentioned in Box 6; types are mentioned in Box 7; and nursing management is mentioned in Box 8.

Box 5: Signs/Symptoms of Personality Disorders

- Persistent, inflexible personality traits.
- Impaired interpersonal relationships.
- Emotional dysregulation (especially in Cluster B disorders).
- Difficulty adapting to social and occupational environments.
- Risk-taking, self-harm, or impulsive behaviors (specific to some types).

Box 6: Risk Factors of Personality Disorders

- Genetic Factors: Family history of mental illness.
- Neurobiological Factors: Brain structure and function abnormalities.
- Environmental Factors: Childhood trauma, neglect, or abuse.
- Social and Cultural Influences: Dysfunctional upbringing or societal pressures.

Box 7: Classification (According to DSM-5)
Personality disorders are categorized into **three clusters** based on similar characteristics:

Cluster A (Odd or Eccentric)
- Paranoid: Distrust and suspicion of others.
- Schizoid: Detachment from social relationships, emotional coldness.
- Schizotypal: Unusual thinking, eccentric behavior, social anxiety.

Cluster B (Dramatic, Emotional, or Erratic)

- Antisocial: Disregard for others' rights, impulsivity, lack of remorse.
- Borderline: Emotional instability, fear of abandonment, impulsive behavior.
- Histrionic: Excessive attention-seeking, emotional overreaction.
- Narcissistic: Grandiosity, need for admiration, lack of empathy.

Cluster C (Anxious or Fearful)

- Avoidant: Extreme social inhibition, sensitivity to criticism.
- Dependent: Excessive need to be taken care of, fear of separation.
- Obsessive-Compulsive: Perfectionism, rigid control, preoccupation with rules.

DSM-5 criteria of personality disorders

- Based on clinical evaluation, psychiatric history, and DSM-5 criteria.
- Symptoms must be long-standing, inflexible, and cause significant distress.

Treatment and Management

- **Psychotherapy (Mainstay of Treatment)**:
  - **Cognitive Behavioral Therapy (CBT)**: Reshapes negative thought patterns.
  - **Dialectical Behavior Therapy (DBT)**: Effective for Borderline PD.
  - **Psychodynamic Therapy**: Explores unconscious conflicts.
- **Medication**: Used for symptom management (e.g., antidepressants, mood stabilizers).
- **Social and Occupational Support**: Helps with functional adaptation.

Box 8: Nursing Management of Personality Disorders

- **Establish Trust**: Use therapeutic communication.
- **Set Clear Boundaries**: Prevent manipulation or dependency.
- **Monitor for Self-Harm**: Especially in Borderline and Antisocial PD.
- **Encourage Adaptive Coping Strategies**: Help develop healthy emotional regulation.
- **Educate Patients and Families**: Reduce stigma, promote treatment adherence.

Differential Diagnosis

Differential diagnosis includes: undiagnosed organic disease, medication side effects, endocrine/metabolic disorders (e.g., thyroid disease), neurological conditions, depressive and anxiety disorders, and factitious disorder. A structured approach minimizes missed medical illness while avoiding excessive testing.

Pathophysiological Mechanisms: An Integrative View

Somatoform phenomena are best understood through a biopsychosocial lens. Mechanisms include heightened interoceptive awareness, central sensitization in pain disorders, dysregulated stress-response systems, and cognitive-affective processes (catastrophizing, attentional bias). Social reinforcement and cultural expressions shape symptom expression.

Management: Principles and Strategies

Management goals include symptom reduction, improved functioning, reduced unnecessary investigations, and enhanced quality of life. Multimodal treatment using pharmacotherapy, psychotherapy, and rehabilitative approaches is evidence-based. A therapeutic alliance and consistent care coordination are central.

5 Medical Management of Somatoform Diseases

Medical management should be conservative, evidence-informed, and patient-centered. Clinicians should aim to minimize iatrogenic harm from excessive testing while ensuring treatable conditions are not overlooked. Shared decision-making and clear treatment plans help align expectations.

Practical Clinical Pathway

A practical pathway includes:

1. Comprehensive history and physical;
2. Targeted investigations guided by red flags;
3. Explanation of findings and proposed plan;
4. Early introduction of psychosocial treatments;
5. Scheduled follow-ups with a primary clinician;
6. Involvement of specialist services when warranted.

1. **General Clinical Approach**

Initial steps include building rapport, validating the patient's experience, conducting a focused diagnostic workup to exclude treatable medical conditions, and setting collaborative goals. Avoid dismissive language; instead emphasize symptom management and functional recovery.

2. **Pharmacological Treatments**

- Selective serotonin reuptake inhibitors (SSRIs) and serotonin norepinephrine reuptake inhibitors (SNRIs) may be effective particularly when depression or anxiety coexists, or when pain-related symptoms are prominent.
- Analgesics and neuropathic pain agents (e.g., duloxetine, gabapentin) can be used judiciously for chronic pain but with careful monitoring for misuse.
- Short-term use of anxiolytics may be considered for acute exacerbations, with caution regarding dependency.

3. **Psychological Interventions**

Evidence-based psychotherapies include Cognitive Behavioral Therapy (CBT), Acceptance and Commitment Therapy (ACT), problem-solving therapy, and interventions targeting stress management and emotion regulation. CBT specifically addresses maladaptive illness beliefs, terrible thinking, and avoidance behaviors.

4. **Collaborative Care and Rehabilitation**

Integrated care models co-locating mental health within primary care improve access and outcomes. Rehabilitation with graded activity, occupational therapy, and physiotherapy supports return to function. Regular single-point primary care follow-up reduces unnecessary specialist referrals and tests.

Nursing Problems and Interventions

Nurses are pivotal in identification, education, care coordination, and delivery of psychotherapeutic and rehabilitative interventions. The following section outlines common nursing diagnoses, goals, and evidence-based interventions with rationales.

1. **Common Nursing Diagnoses**

Common nursing diagnoses include:

- Anxiety related to perceived serious illness.
- Ineffective coping related to maladaptive health behaviors.
- Activity intolerance related to fatigue and pain.
- Social isolation related to chronic illness behavior and role withdrawal.
- Deficient knowledge regarding psychosomatic nature of symptoms and management strategies.

2. **Nursing Care Plan and Interventions**

Below are examples of nursing problems, measurable goals, and interventions that can be adapted to local settings. Interventions emphasize therapeutic communication, education, behavioral activation, and coordination with multidisciplinary teams.

Anxiety related to perceived serious illness

Goal: Patient will demonstrate reduced anxiety (self-report) and decreased excessive health-related behaviors within 4 weeks.

Nursing interventions:

1. Establish a trusting therapeutic relationship; use open-ended questions and active listening.
2. Provide clear, simple explanations of diagnostic findings and the rationale for recommended care.
3. Teach anxiety reduction techniques (deep breathing, progressive muscle relaxation, guided imagery).
4. Develop a structured appointment schedule to reduce unscheduled visits and reassurance seeking.

Ineffective coping related to maladaptive illness beliefs

Goal: Patient will identify at least two adaptive coping strategies and use them in response to symptom flare-ups.

Nursing interventions:

1. Assess coping style and existing resources.
2. Provide psychoeducation about the mind–body connection and role of stress in symptom strengthening.
3. Collaborate with psychology services to initiate CBT or problem-solving therapy.
4. Encourage journaling to identify triggers and patterns.

Activity intolerance related to chronic pain and fatigue

Goal: Patient will engage in graded activity program and increase daily activity tolerance by 20% over 6 weeks.

Nursing interventions:

1. Implement a graded exercise or activity plan in collaboration with physiotherapy.
2. Set realistic, measurable activity goals and celebrate incremental progress.
3. Educate on energy conservation techniques and pacing.
4. Monitor for signs of overexertion and adjust plan accordingly.

Deficient knowledge regarding condition and treatment

Goal: Patient will correctly describe the nature of their disorder and two self-management strategies within 2 teaching sessions.

Nursing interventions:

1. Provide tailored educational materials (written and verbal) at appropriate literacy level.
2. Use teach-back method to confirm understanding.
3. Involve family members in education sessions to align expectations and reduce reinforcement of sick role.
4. Refer to peer support groups or community resources.

Communication Strategies and Therapeutic Alliance

Effective communication is central. Strategies include validating the patient's symptoms, avoiding premature psychiatric labeling, and naming the mind–body connection in non-judgmental terms (e.g., 'I believe your symptoms are real, and stress can make symptoms worse'). Establishing structured follow-up appointments and using consistent messaging across clinicians reduces patient anxiety and unnecessary medical utilization.

Documentation and Legal/Ethical Considerations

Accurate documentation of symptom chronology, investigations, explanations given, and patient education is essential. Ethical care requires respect for patient's experiences while avoiding reinforcement of maladaptive illness behaviors. When capacity or safety is a concern (e.g., severe suicidality, functional decline), escalate to appropriate services promptly.

Outcome Evaluation and Follow-Up

Outcome measures include symptom severity scales, functional assessments (ADLs, occupational participation), quality-of-life indices, and healthcare utilization metrics. Nursing follow-up should track progress against goals, adherence to therapeutic plans, and early signals of relapse or comorbid psychiatric illness.

Case Picture

Ms. A, a 34-year-old woman, presents with six months of intermittent chest pain, fatigue, and dizziness. Extensive cardiac workup was normal. She reports high stress at work and difficulty sleeping. She frequently visits multiple specialists seeking reassurance. A collaborative approach involving primary care, psychiatry, and nursing resulted in the diagnosis of Somatic Symptom Disorder. The care plan included CBT referral, SSRI for comorbid anxiety, graded exercise, and scheduled primary care follow-ups. Over 12 weeks, her symptom preoccupation reduced, activity increased, and emergency visits declined.

Take Home Message

- Somatoform and psychosomatic disorders are common, disabling, and medically challenging.
- Contemporary classification emphasizes symptom burden and maladaptive health-related behaviors.
- A biopsychosocial framework guides diagnosis and management.
- Nurses play a central role in assessment, education, care coordination, and delivery of behavioral interventions.
- Integrated, patient-centered approaches reduce unnecessary investigations and improve function.

Sample Short Answer Questions

1. What is the main difference between Somatic Symptom Disorder and Illness Anxiety Disorder?
2. Name two important risk factors that can make someone more likely to develop a somatoform disorder.
3. What is one main goal when treating a patient with a somatoform disorder?

Sample Essay Questions

1. How can stress and emotions cause real physical sickness?

2. If a patient is worried about unexplained physical symptoms, what is the best way for a nurse to help them?
3. Explain the role of a nurse in managing a patient with a somatoform disorder, listing two specific nursing interventions and their rationales.

1 A core principle for managing these disorders is to:			2. Somatic symptom disorder focus		
	(a)	Order every possible test for reassurance	F	(a)	• Focuses on proving symptoms are fake
✓	(b)	Build a consistent, trusting patient relationship	T	(b)	• Requires symptoms for over 6 months
	(c)	Tell the patient the pain isn't real	T	(c)	Emphasizes the patient's excessive worry about symptoms
	(d)	Focus only on medication	T	(d)	• Can be diagnosed even if a medical cause is found
			F	(e)	• Is the same as illness anxiety disorder?

Suggested Reading

American Psychiatric Association. (2013). *Diagnostic and statistical manual of mental disorders* (5th ed.).

Fink, P., & Schröder, A. (2010). One single diagnosis, bodily distress syndrome, succeeded to capture 10 diagnostic categories of functional somatic syndromes and somatoform disorders. *Journal of Psychosomatic Research, 68*(5), 415–426. https://doi.org/10.1016/j.jpsychores.2010.02.004

Kirmayer, L. J., & Looper, K. J. (2006). Abnormal illness behaviour: Physiological, psychological and social dimensions of somatoform and related disorders. *Social Science & Medicine, 62*(3), 531–542. https://doi.org/10.1016/j.socscimed.2005.06.020

Mayou, R., Kirmayer, L. J., Simon, G., Kroenke, K., & Sharpe, M. (2005). Somatoform disorders: Time for a new approach in DSM-V. *American Journal of Psychiatry, 162*(5), 847–855. https://doi.org/10.1176/appi.ajp.162.5.847

Rief, W., & Martin, A. (2014). How to use the new DSM-5 somatic symptom disorder diagnosis in research and practice: A critical evaluation and a proposal for modifications. *Psychosomatic Medicine, 76*(4), 422–427. https://doi.org/10.1097/PSY.0000000000000077

World Health Organization (WHO). (2022). *International Classification of Diseases, 11th Revision (ICD-11): Clinical descriptions and diagnostic guidelines for mental, behavioural or neurodevelopmental disorders*. WHO.

Chapter 9
Care of Clients with Neuropsychiatric Disorders: Obsessive–Compulsive Disorder

Sultana Algin and S. M. Yasir Arafat

Abstract Obsessive–Compulsive Disorder (OCD) is a chronic and debilitating neuropsychiatric disorder characterized by the presence of obsessions, compulsions, or both. The prevalence of OCD was 0.5% among adults and 1.3% among children and adolescents in Bangladesh. A combination of genetics, temperament, and life stressors can trigger OCD in susceptible individuals. Genetic and environmental factors are responsible for OCD. Pharmacological agents, psychotherapy, and social rehabilitation are major management ways. Nursing management of OCD can be life-changing for the patients. It aims to provide holistic care to the patients, addressing both their psychological and physiological needs. This chapter discusses epidemiology, clinical features, etiology, and medical and nursing management of OCD in Bangladesh perspective.

Keywords Neuropsychiatric disorder · Obsessive–compulsive disorder · OCD · Bangladesh · Psychiatric nursing

Obsessive–Compulsive Disorder (OCD) is a neuropsychiatric disorder that is prevalent across the world. It is often a hidden misery that causes lifelong suffering. Early in the twentieth century, the groundbreaking work of psychiatrists Sigmund Freud and Pierre Janet helped to establish our current knowledge of OCD. Freud coined the word "Zwangsneurose" to characterize the symptoms he saw in patients who were struggling with obsession and/or compulsion. Later, the word was translated as "obsession" in New York and "compulsion" in London. Eventually, a compromise between the two languages led to the condition being referred to as "obsessive–compulsive." The *Diagnostic and Statistical Manual of Mental Disorders, Fifth Edition* (DSM 5) includes Body Dysmorphic Disorder (BDD), Hoarding Disorder,

S. Algin
Department of Psychiatry, Bangladesh Medical University, Dhaka, Bangladesh

S. M. Y. Arafat (✉)
Department of Psychiatry, Bangladesh Specialized Hospital, Dhaka, Bangladesh
e-mail: arafatdmc62@gmail.com

S. M. Y. Arafat and H. Akter (eds.), *Psychiatric Nursing in Bangladesh*, Mental Health Systems and Policy in Low- and Middle-Income Countries,
https://doi.org/10.1007/978-981-95-8501-4_9

Trichotillomania (Hair-Pulling Disorder), Excoriation (Skin-Picking) Disorder in the OCD-related spectrum.

According to the World Health Organization, among those aged 15 to 44 years, OCD ranks among the top 20 causes of illness-based disability worldwide. Men and women get OCD at about the same rate. People of various colors, ethnicities, and backgrounds also have about the same prevalence of OCD. It can start during any age; however, the onset of symptoms usually happens in late adolescence or early adulthood, or between the ages of 8 and 12 years. The rate usually varies from 0.5% to 3% among adults in the community. The prevalence of OCD was 0.5% among adults and 1.3% among children and adolescents in Bangladesh.

1 Sign/Symptoms

OCD is a chronic and debilitating neuropsychiatric disorder characterized by the presence of obsessions, compulsions, or both.

- **Obsessions** are recurrent, persistent, intrusive, and unwanted, irrational thoughts, urges or images that cause significant anxiety and distress. The person wants to ignore, suppress, or try to neutralize them with some other thought or action.
- **Compulsions** are repetitive behaviors or mental acts that individual feels driven to perform in response to obsession (thoughts, urges, or images) or according to rules that must be applied rigidly and aimed at preventing or reducing anxiety or distress or preventing dreaded event or situation.

DSM-5 Diagnostic Criteria for OCD

A. **Presence of obsessions, compulsions, or both:**

1. **Obsessions** are defined by both:
   - Recurrent and persistent thoughts, urges, or images that are experienced as intrusive and unwanted, and that in most individuals cause marked anxiety or distress.
   - The individual attempts to ignore or suppress such thoughts, urges, or images, or to neutralize them with some other thought or action (e.g., by performing a compulsion).

2. **Compulsions** are defined by both:
   - Repetitive behaviors (e.g., hand washing, ordering, checking) or mental acts (e.g., praying, counting, repeating words silently) that the individual feels driven to perform in response to an obsession or according to rules that must be applied rigidly.

- The behaviors or mental acts are aimed at preventing or reducing anxiety or distress, or preventing some dreaded event or situation; however, these behaviors or mental acts are not connected in a realistic way with what they are designed to neutralize or prevent, or they are clearly excessive.

B. **The obsessions or compulsions are time-consuming** (e.g., take more than 1 h per day) or cause clinically significant distress or impairment in social, occupational, or other important areas of functioning.
C. **The obsessive–compulsive symptoms are not attributable to the physiological effects of a substance** (e.g., a drug of abuse, a medication) or another medical condition.
D. **The disturbance is not better explained by the symptoms of another mental disorder,** such as:

- Excessive worries (as in Generalized Anxiety Disorder)
- Preoccupation with appearance (as in Body Dysmorphic Disorder)
- Difficulty discarding or parting with possessions (as in Hoarding Disorder)
- Ritualized eating behavior (as in Eating Disorders)
- Recurrent sexual urges or fantasies (as in Paraphilic Disorders), etc.

Specifiers

1. **With good or fair insight:** The individual recognizes that OCD beliefs are definitely or probably not true, or that they may or may not be true.
2. **With poor insight:** The individual thinks OCD beliefs are probably true.
3. **With absent insight/delusional beliefs:** The individual is completely convinced that OCD beliefs are true.
4. **Tic-related:** The individual has a current or past history of a tic disorder.

Each OCD case is unique, and individuals with OCD have a cluster of symptoms that might vary in intensity. The symptoms can include obsessive thoughts and compulsions of different dimensions about a particular issue, theme, or concern, and duties, differing from person to person and culture to culture.

A vicious cycle goes on in which distress and anxiety are brought on by obsession. They repress or neutralize their thoughts or engage in safety behaviors to feel comfortable and relieved. Once more, obsessions and compulsions recur when triggering factors are present until the patient's anxiety and anguish are alleviated (Fig. 1).

Obsessional thoughts are noted in various presentations like dirt and contamination, harm-related obsession, religious, sexual, pathological doubts, needs for symmetry/exactness, hoarding, and miscellaneous. Compulsions are presented in various ways, like cleaning, checking, counting, mental acts, avoidance behavior, rituals/repeated behaviors, hoarding, and miscellaneous. OCD is a disorder with high comorbidity of psychiatric disorders; 76% have a lifetime history of another anxiety disorder, such

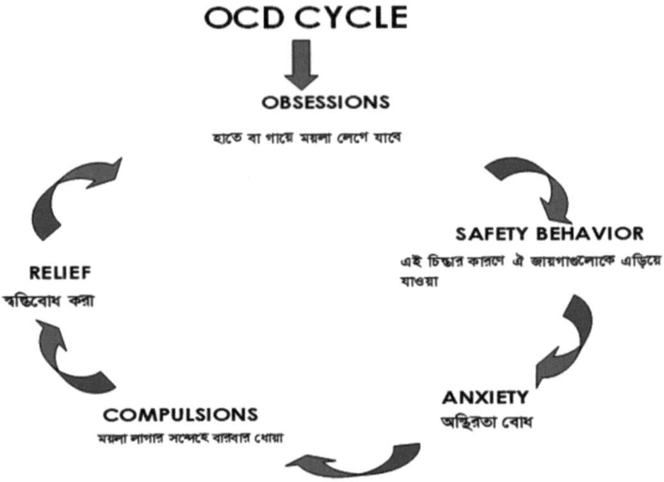
OCD CYCLE
OBSESSIONS
হাতে বা গায়ে ময়লা লেগে যাবে
SAFETY BEHAVIOR
এই চিন্তার কারণে ঐ জায়গাগুলোকে এড়িয়ে যাওয়া
ANXIETY
অস্থিরতা বোধ
COMPULSIONS
ময়লা লাগার সন্দেহে বারবার ধোয়া
RELIEF
স্বস্তিবোধ করা

Fig. 1 The OCD cycle

as panic disorder, social anxiety disorder, generalized anxiety disorder, or a specific phobia, 63% have a lifetime history of a mood disorder—the most common is major depressive disorder, 23% to 32% have coexisting obsessive–compulsive personality disorder, and up to 29% of individuals with OCD seeking treatment have a lifetime history of a tic disorder.

Risk Factors for OCD

A combination of genetics, temperament, and life stressors can trigger OCD in susceptible individuals. Genetic and environmental factors are responsible for OCD. In addition, psychological factors play as maintenance factors (Fig. 2, Box 1,2). While it is difficult to determine the exact cause of OCD, experts believe several risk factors make a person more likely to develop this condition.

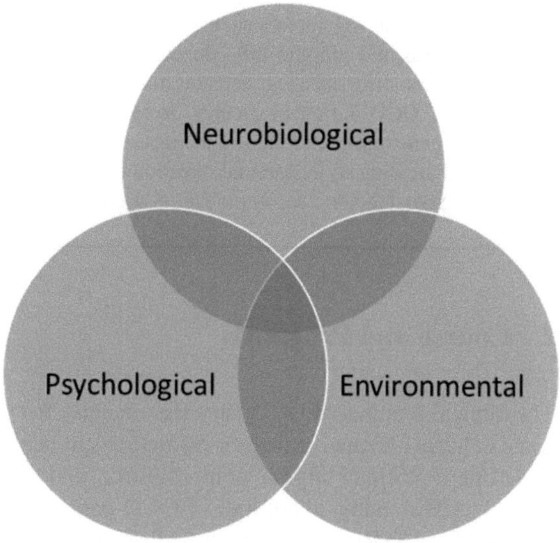

Fig. 2 Risk factor domains of OCD

Box 1: Risk Factors for OCD

1. Neurobiological Factors
   a. Genetics—Polygenic
   b. Family history—Having a first-degree relative (parent, sibling, or child) with OCD significantly increases the risk of developing the disorder. Symptoms appearing during childhood or adolescence may suggest a higher genetic and familial contribution.
   c. Brain structure—abnormalities in several brain regions and circuits, primarily involving the orbitofrontal cortex, anterior cingulate cortex (ACC), striatum (including the caudate nucleus and putamen), and thalamus.
   d. Biochemical abnormalities—Dysregulation of Serotonin, Dopamine, GABA, and Glutamate.
2. Psychological Factors
   a. Psychodynamic factor—secondary gains.
   b. Interpersonal dimension—relatives accommodate the patient through active participation in rituals or significant modifications of daily routines.
   c. In psychoanalytic theory—regression from oedipal phase to anal psychosexual phase of development.
   d. The coexistence of love and hatred toward the same person leaves the patient with doubt and indecisions (ambivalence).
3. Environmental Factors
   a. Streptococcal infection, head injury, stressful life events

b. Prenatal risk factors such as maternal smoking during pregnancy, premature birth, and complications during labor and delivery.
c. Hormonal changes: females may be susceptible to developing symptoms of OCD during pregnancy or postpartum, as well as after beginning their menstrual cycles, during menopause, or following a miscarriage.
d. Parenting style: parental rejection or parental overprotection
e. Social factors: accommodation, social isolation, lower rates of marriage

2 Course and Prognosis

The clinical features of OCD vary significantly from culture to culture as there are some cultural affirmative factors. Sometimes, it takes many years to reach a psychiatrist due to societal stigma, comorbidities, underdiagnoses, and a subpar referral system. Additionally, about half of OCD patients had never gotten an appropriate dosage of an SSRI, one in seven had received improper medications, and almost one-third had never received any pharmacotherapy.

In the case of OCD, two major types of course are seen—chronic and episodic. A chronic course implies a near-persistent presence of symptoms. Symptom severity might wax and wane, with phasic exacerbations and incomplete remissions; however, there is never a complete relief from symptoms. In episodic course, symptoms are present only during an episode, and for the remaining time, symptoms remit, with or without treatment.

Across OCD studies, there is significant variability in reported predictors. Sociodemographic variables, illness characteristics, and comorbid disorders have all been identified as prognostic factors. The most consistent of these include—age at onset, baseline illness severity and duration, and early treatment response. Early recognition and detection of these issues may help to intervene in OCD. These factors are considered while formulating the management plan (Table 1).

Table 1 Risk and protective factors for OCD

Predisposing factor	Family history (genetic loading), early life experience, pattern of parenting, personality, high expressed emotion (HEE) or low expressed emotion (LEE-criticism, hostility, emotional over involvement)
Precipitating factor	Recent life events (adverse/loss events/threat events), environmental stress, effects of physical illness
Perpetuating factor (Maintaining factor)	Avoidance, safety behavior, family accommodation, HEE or LEE family, self-harm, substance abuse, non-compliance to treatment, comorbidity (Chronic medical illness and/or psychiatric illness)
Protective factor	Good insight, drug compliance, supportive family, financial solvency, employment

Box 2: Cultural affirmative factors for OCD

- Muslims: religious matters related to cleanliness and dirt
- South America: Aggressive obsession
- USA: Dirt and contamination obsession
- The Indian and British: mostly related to orderliness and aggressive issues
- Jews: Emphasis on cleanliness and orderliness

Box 3: Management Approach for OCD

Biological

- Pharmacological
- Psychosurgery and newer brain stimulation techniques

Psychological

- Psychoeducation
- CBT-based ERP
- Mindfulness
- Acceptance Commitment Therapy (ACT)

Social

- Ensure drug compliance and psychotherapy
- Move to active daily life program

Medical Management of OCD

The **medical management of OCD** primarily involves the use of pharmacological treatments, combined with psychotherapy, to alleviate symptoms and improve the patient's quality of life (Box 3). Here's an overview of the key components:

1. **Pharmacological Treatment**
    - **Selective Serotonin Reuptake Inhibitors (SSRIs)**
        - **First-Line Treatment**: SSRIs are the most commonly prescribed medications for OCD due to their efficacy in reducing symptoms.
        - **Examples**: Fluoxetine, Sertraline, Fluvoxamine, Escitalopram.
        - **Dosage**: Often higher than those used for depression and requires several weeks to show improvement.

- **Tricyclic Antidepressants (TCAs)**
  - **Clomipramine**: This TCA is particularly effective for OCD, though it has more side effects compared to SSRIs.

- **Augmentation Strategies**
  - **Antipsychotics**: In cases where SSRIs are not fully effective, antipsychotics like Risperidone or Aripiprazole may be used as augmentative therapy.

- **Other Medications**
  - **SNRIs (Serotonin-Norepinephrine Reuptake Inhibitors)**: Like Venlafaxine, sometimes used if SSRIs are ineffective.
  - **Benzodiazepines**: Occasionally prescribed for short-term relief of acute anxiety, though not recommended for long-term use due to the risk of dependency.

2. **Psychotherapy:** could be individual or group approach
   - **Psychoeducation:** It is an early intervention and plays a vital role in the destigmatization. This educational process includes up-to-date information about the illness, treatment options, and how to monitor symptoms and prevent relapse.
   - **Cognitive-Behavioral Therapy (CBT)**:
     - **Exposure and Response Prevention (ERP)**: A key component of CBT, ERP involves gradually exposing the patient to anxiety-provoking situations while preventing compulsive responses.
   - **Acceptance and Commitment Therapy (ACT)**: ACT-based exposure is similar to ERP (Exposure and Response Prevention) but shifts the focus from reducing anxiety to increasing willingness to experience discomfort while engaging in valued actions.
   - **Family Therapy**:
     - Helps involve family members in the treatment process, providing education and strategies to support the patient and reduce family stress.
3. **Social Rehabilitation:** Encourage the patient to participate actively in a daily life program while ensuring drug compliance and psychotherapy. Inform family members about family accommodation.
4. **Lifestyle and Supportive Measures**
   - Stress Management: Techniques such as mindfulness, meditation, and relaxation exercises can help reduce overall anxiety levels.
   - Healthy Lifestyle: Encouraging regular physical activity, serotonin rich food, adequate sunlight exposure, sleep about 6-7 h, drink adequate water.

5. **Monitoring and Follow-Up:**
   - Regular Assessment: Monitoring for medication side effects, effectiveness, and adherence is crucial.
   - Adjusting Treatment: Based on the patient's response, the treatment plan may need modifications, including changes in medication or therapy focus.

Nursing Problems and Interventions for OCD

Obsessive–Compulsive Disorder is a debilitating condition that requires early intervention and better supportive services. If neglected for long, it can affect personal, social, and professional life. Nursing care can help patients with OCD in management with their understanding and appropriate care. There are different presentation of obsession and compulsion that causes anxiety and distress among the patient. Even they attempted deliberate self-harm, suicide attempt to remove, suppress or neutralize those obsessions by compulsive behavior. A nursing diagnosis for OCD identifies specific problems that a patient with OCD is suffering from. These diagnoses help patients receive nursing interventions to address the issues. Nursing diagnosis for OCD:

1. Anxiety (Related to Obsessive Thoughts and Compulsions)

Evidence: The patient shows signs of excessive worry, intrusive thoughts, and compulsive ritualistic behaviors.

Nursing Interventions:

The nurse involves the patient in deep breathing exercises and mindfulness techniques to promote calmness.
Talk to the patient to reassure them and provide emotional support.
Show the patient the triggers that cause the compulsive behavior.
Teach coping mechanisms to help the patient deal with OCD symptoms.

2. Impaired Social Interaction (Related to Repetitive Behaviors and Social Withdrawal)

Evidence: The patient avoids social gatherings and is having difficulty in all types of relationships.

Nursing Interventions:

A nurse can help the patient accept gradual exposure to social situations.
Provide structured therapy sessions for improved interpersonal skills.
Encourage the patient to participate in group therapy or support groups.

3. Ineffective Coping (Related to Compulsive Rituals and Obsessive Thoughts)

Evidence: The patient continues to feel overwhelmed and performs rituals to reduce anxiety while struggling to control compulsive behavior.

Nursing Interventions:

Guide with cognitive restructuring by teaching alternative coping mechanisms.
Provide ERP therapy to gradually reduce compulsive reactions to triggers.
Show the patient stress management techniques to deal with anxiety effectively.

4. Sleep Pattern Disturbance (Related to Intrusive Thoughts and Anxiety)

Evidence: The patient finds it difficult to fall or stay asleep because of obsessive thinking.

Nursing Interventions:

Guiding and promoting good sleep hygiene practices.
Helping patients to learn and practice relaxation techniques before bedtime for better sleep quality.
Therapy sessions and daily routines to address underlying reasons for anxiety relief.

5. Risk for Self-Harm (Related to Distress and Depression Associated with OCD)

Evidence: The patient has thoughts of self-harm and suicide due to immense emotional distress.

Nursing Interventions:

Regular assessment to check self-harm tendencies and suicidal thoughts.
Intervene to manage crises and provide mental support.
Provide the patient with therapies and counseling to understand and address the cause and depressive thoughts.

Nursing Management of OCD

Nursing management of OCD can be life-changing for the patients. It aims to provide holistic care to the patients, addressing both their psychological and physiological needs. The comprehensive attention aids with the overall well-being of the patient, showing improvement in symptoms and mental health.

Nursing Management of OCD

1. **Assessment and Monitoring**

   Thorough Evaluation: Conduct a detailed psychiatric assessment of the patient using psychiatric assessment tools (History taking sheet, Y-BOCS, DOCS-B).

Identify Triggers: The behavior patterns are observed regularly to identify triggers.

The patients are monitored for their response to the treatment and nursing intervention.

2. **Building a Therapeutic Relationship**

   - **Establish Trust**: Develop rapport with the patient to encourage open communication and reduce feelings of shame or embarrassment about their symptoms.
   - **Provide Emotional Support**: Offer reassurance and empathy to help the patient feel understood and supported.

3. **Psychoeducation**

   - **Educate the Patient and Family**: Explain OCD, its nature, and the treatment options, including the role of medication and therapy.
   - **Normalize Experiences**: Help the patient understand that OCD is a treatable condition and that they are not alone in their experiences.

4. **Encourage Therapy Participation**

   - **Cognitive-Behavioral Therapy (CBT)**: Support participation in CBT, especially Exposure and Response Prevention (ERP), which is a key therapeutic approach for OCD.
   - **Regular Therapy Sessions**: Encourage consistent attendance in therapy sessions to address and gradually reduce symptoms.

5. **Medication Management**

   - Manage dosage and adherence to prescription medicines used for anxiety in patients.
   - The response and side effects are both monitored.
   - The patient is educated about the expected effects of the medicine and how and why to adhere to the doses.

6. **Stress Management and Coping Skills**

   - **Teach Relaxation Techniques**: Introduce methods such as deep breathing, mindfulness, and progressive muscle relaxation to help manage anxiety.
   - **Develop Healthy Coping Strategies**: Encourage the patient to use positive coping mechanisms instead of compulsive behaviors.

7. **Safety and Environment**

   Make a customized structured routine to.

   - ensure exercise, meditation, nutrition, work, and other activities without much exposure to things that increase anxiety, to minimize it.
   - involve the family members to encourage the patient to follow the routine successfully and ensure a non-judgmental and understanding environment.

8. **Encouraging Self-Care and Independence**
    - Teaching patients to manage their own routine and daily tasks without following any ritualistic behavior.
    - Support them with gradual exposure of triggers to manage their symptoms and increase their threshold.
9. **Involvement of Family**
    - **Family Support**: Involve family members in the treatment process and educate them on how to support the patient effectively.
    - **Family Therapy**: Consider family therapy sessions to improve family dynamics and understanding of the disorder.
10. **Documentation and Continuous Evaluation**
    - **Record Progress**: Keep detailed records of the patient's progress, changes in symptoms, and responses to treatment.
    - **Reevaluate Care Plan**: Regularly review and adjust the care plan based on the patient's evolving needs and treatment response.

Case Discussion

Sumon, a 24-year-old unmarried male, came with his parents with the complaints of recurrent intrusive blasphemous thoughts, fear of committing suicide, compulsive praying, and avoidance behaviors for 4–5 years. He had recurrent intrusive thoughts related to harming others, excessive reassurance-seeking, and checking behaviors. His mother mentioned his sadness, hopelessness, fatigue, and excessive worry about academic performance and future that increased over the last few days. Sumon stated that for the past 4–5 years, he has experienced distressing, repetitive, and intrusive thoughts that he identifies as blasphemous. These thoughts include mental images of insulting God or religious figures, especially while praying or reading the Qur'an. He described being overwhelmed with guilt and fear that he may unintentionally commit a grave sin or be punished. As a result, he often repeats his prayers, washes himself before every prayer multiple times, and avoids religious gatherings for fear he might do something wrong again. He sometimes thought about committing suicide as he couldn't get rid of such distressing thought. He also taps certain objects in a fixed number, seeking reassurance from family that he's a "good person." Parents initially couldn't accept this as a disorder; they physically, verbally, and emotionally insulted and criticized him. Now he feels hopeless, fatigue, and excessive worry about career and future that increased for few days. This is the first time he visited a psychiatrist.

Personally, he is an introvert, a polite person, has few friends, talks with them over mobile, and stays away from social events. He is the first among his three siblings. His father is a banker and also had obsessive symptoms like checking counting. His early childhood was not significant. Up until class VII, he was an excellent student;

after that, his academic performance steadily declined. After that, such symptoms progressively impacted his daily, social, professional, and academic pursuits. He began smoking a few months ago.

On mental state examination (MSE), his mood was found to be depressed and had suicidal ideation. The obsession-blasphemous thought, image, harm-related obsession, and compulsion—mental prayer, avoidance of sharp objects, and repeated asking for assurance—were sorted out. There were no perceptual symptoms or cognitive deficits found. Insight was good.

Sumon meets the criteria of obsessive–compulsive disorder (according to DSM-5). He acknowledged that these thoughts and compulsions originated from his own mind and that they were unreasonable, irrational. He made an effort to stifle the thought at first, but ultimately he was unable to do so. There are a few depressive symptoms secondary to obsessions and compulsions that do not meet the criteria of a depressive episode.

3 Management

After doing routine investigations and severity assessment, treatment plan was followed. Psychoeducation about disorder to patient and his family. Explained and ensured about the importance to follow biopsychosocial approach. Pharmacological: Fluvoxamine started at 50 mg/day, titrated to 150 mg/day (any SSRI could be tried) and ensured regular follow-up. Exposer and response prevention was suggested along with family education to intervene critical comments from the parents specially. Good insight and absence of psychotic features predict better outcomes.

Take Home Message

- OCD is generally considered to be a lifelong condition affecting males and females equally across the world.
- The prevalence of OCD was 0.5% among adults and 1.3% among children and adolescents in Bangladesh.
- Symptoms comprise either obsessions or compulsions, or in combination.
- It is treatable; treatment reduces the symptoms and improves the quality of life.
- Biopsychosocial measures are well-accepted methods of management.

Sample Short Answer Questions

1. Define obsession or compulsion.
2. What is Obsessive–Compulsive Disorder?
3. What are the common features of obsessions or compulsions?
4. Mention the risk factors/etiology/causes and signs & symptoms of OCD.

Sample Essay Questions

1. Discuss the DSM-5 Diagnostic Criteria for OCD.
2. Describe the medical management of OCD.
3. As a psychiatric nurse, how will you manage a case of OCD in your ward?

Sample Multiple Choice Questions (MCQs) and Best Answer Question

Nursing Problems in Obsessive–Compulsive Disorder involve-			Which intervention is effective for managing OCD?		
T	a)	Anxiety is common in OCD		a)	Ignoring symptoms
F	b)	OCD requires nursing interventions	✓	b)	Cognitive-behavioral therapy
T	c)	Social functioning is often impaired		c)	Avoiding discussions about compulsions
F	d)	Clients aren't always aware of compulsions		d)	Solely relying on medication
T	e)	Self-harm risk may exist in severe cases			

Suggested Reading

Abramowitz, J. S., Taylor, S., & McKay, D. (2009). Obsessive-compulsive disorder. *Lancet, 374*(9688), 491–499. https://doi.org/10.1016/S0140-6736(09)60240-3

Cervin, M. (2023). Obsessive-compulsive disorder: Diagnosis, clinical features, nosology, and epidemiology. *The Psychiatric clinics of North America, 46*(1), 1–16. https://doi.org/10.1016/j.psc.2022.10.006

Grant, J. E. (2014). Clinical practice: Obsessive-compulsive disorder. *The New England Journal of Medicine, 371*(7), 646–653. https://doi.org/10.1056/NEJMcp1402176

Stein, D. J., Costa, D. L. C., Lochner, C., Miguel, E. C., Reddy, Y. C. J., Shavitt, R. G., van den Heuvel, O. A., & Simpson, H. B. (2019). Obsessive-compulsive disorder. Nature reviews. *Disease Primers, 5*(1), 52. https://doi.org/10.1038/s41572-019-0102-3

Chapter 10
Care of Clients with Delirium, Dementia, and Other Related Disorders

Redwana Hossain and S. M. Yasir Arafat

Abstract Delirium and dementia are the most prevalent neurocognitive disorders, both characterized by impaired cognitive functioning but distinguished by the presence of altered consciousness in delirium and progressive forgetfulness in dementia. Delirium is an acute, fluctuating disturbance in attention and awareness, often precipitated by medical illness, polypharmacy, or environmental factors, common in hospitalized and terminally ill patients. Dementia, or major neurocognitive disorder, is a progressive decline in multiple cognitive domains without disturbance of consciousness, most frequently caused by Alzheimer's disease, vascular pathology, or Lewy body disease. Risk factors for both disorders include modifiable and non-modifiable factors. Management of neurocognitive disorders involves identifying underlying causes, providing supportive care, and implementing individualized non-pharmacological and pharmacological interventions. Nursing care focuses on maintaining safety, promoting orientation, supporting basic needs, addressing behavioral and psychological symptoms, and providing caregiver education. Early detection and comprehensive, multidisciplinary management of delirium and dementia can improve outcomes and quality of life for affected individuals and their families.

Keywords Neuropsychiatric disorder · Delirium · Dementia · Neurocognitive disorder · Bangladesh · Psychiatric nursing

Cognition is a mental process involving perception, attention, memory, learning, executive functioning, language, problem-solving, and decision-making. When cognitive dysfunction arises, it impairs the daily functioning of the person, depending on the area of cognition affected. Delirium and dementia are the most prevalent neurocognitive disorders. Both disorders affect the cognitive process; however, the

---

R. Hossain
Department of Psychiatry, Shaheed Suhrawardy Medical College Hospital, Dhaka, Bangladesh

S. M. Y. Arafat (✉)
Department of Psychiatry, Bangladesh Specialized Hospital, Dhaka, Bangladesh
e-mail: arafatdmc62@gmail.com

S. M. Y. Arafat and H. Akter (eds.), *Psychiatric Nursing in Bangladesh*, Mental Health Systems and Policy in Low- and Middle-Income Countries,
https://doi.org/10.1007/978-981-95-8501-4_10

core distinguishing feature is alteration of consciousness, which is observed in delirium but not in dementia, where prolonged forgetfulness is the key.

1 Definition of Delirium

Delirium is a disturbance in cognitive function reflected as a global impairment of consciousness leading to reduced level of alertness, attention, and perception of the environment. There are other synonymous terms for delirium, including acute confusional state, acute organic syndrome, acute cerebral insufficiency, acute global cognitive dysfunction, altered mental state, and confusion. However, delirium is the preferred diagnostic term both in *the Diagnostic and Statistical Manual of Mental Disorders* (DSM-5) and the *International Classification of Diseases* (ICD-11).

2 DSM-5 Diagnostic Criteria for Delirium

A. A disturbance in attention (i.e., reduced ability to direct, focus, sustain, and shift attention) and awareness (reduced orientation to the environment).
B. The disturbance develops over a short period of time (usually hours to a few days), represents a change from baseline attention and awareness, and tends to fluctuate in severity during the course of a day.
C. An additional disturbance in cognition (e.g., memory deficit, disorientation, language, visuospatial ability, or perception).
D. The disturbance in criteria A and C is not better explained by another neurocognitive disorder and does not occur in the context of severely reduced levels of arousal, such as coma.
E. There is evidence from the history, physical examination, or laboratory findings that the disturbance is a direct physiological consequence of another medical condition, substance intoxication or withdrawal (i.e., due to a drug of abuse or to a medication), or exposure to a toxin, or is due to multiple etiologies.

The delirium can further be specified by duration (acute vs. persistent), level of psychomotor activity (hyperactive, hypoactive, and mixed) and substance intoxication/withdrawal/medication-induced/another medical condition/multiple etiologies delirium.

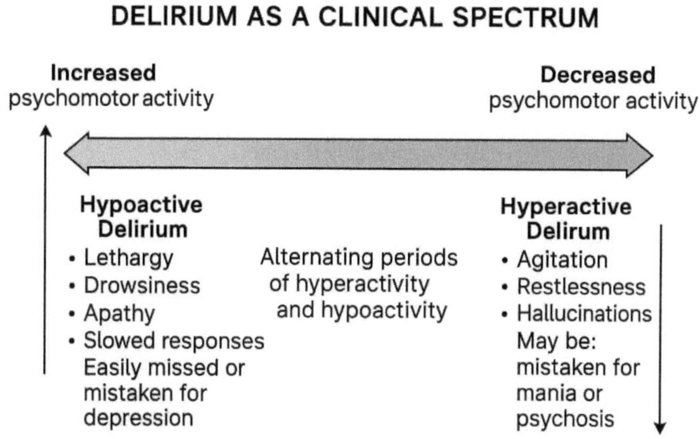

Fig. 1 Delirium as a clinical spectrum

3 Signs/Symptoms of Delirium

The core feature of delirium is an altered level of consciousness. Fluctuations over a 24-h period and reversal of sleep–wake cycle are very common. Other sign-symptoms vary widely between patients depending on the time of day (worse at night) and underlying cause. Symptoms may range from agitation, restlessness, and irritability to lethargy, drowsiness, and slowed response (Fig. 1). Delusions (e.g., persecutory and referential) and hallucinations (visual, tactile, and auditory) may present but not in well well-elaborated form.

Along with inattention and disorientation, visuospatial disturbance, memory deficits, psychomotor retardation and agitation, perceptual disturbance from illusion to hallucinations, language disturbance, thought process abnormalities, and affect lability are other important clinical presentations.

4 Epidemiology

Delirium is most prevalent in specialized hospital settings such as postoperative, intensive care, and palliative care settings. Emergency department and general medical ward also has to deal with delirious patient in a significant number. The prevalence ranges from 6 to 56% in general hospital which might be as much as 90% in terminally ill patients. In community setting, the overall prevalence is only 1–2%.

Table 1 Risk factors of delirium

Modifiable	• Pain, emotional distress • Instrumentation, restraints • Medication, polypharmacy • Biochemical abnormalities • Dehydration • Infections
Potentially modifiable	• Sensory impairment • Immobilization • Substance abuse • Acute severe illness; malnutrition
Non-modifiable	• Age > 65 years • Male sex • Cognitive impairment; history of delirium • History of depression • Comorbidity burden, surgery • Terminal illness

5 Risk Factors for Delirium

Delirium is more predominant in geriatric population and often multifactorial. Precipitating factors in predisposed individual are most vulnerable factor for development of delirium. It is evident that highly vulnerable population develop delirium with minor precipitant like urinary tract infection whereas less vulnerable people need more noxious stimuli (e.g., severe sepsis) to develop delirium.

The most important risk factor for delirium is preexisting neurocognitive disorder (e.g., dementia). Common risk factors are classified in literature under three broad dimensions—predisposing (non-modifiable), precipitating (modifiable), and perpetuating (potentially modifiable). Table 1 shows the common risk factors of development of delirium.

6 Medical Management of Delirium

Delirium is preventable as the risk factors are well established. Pharmacological and non-pharmacological strategies are recommended for both prevention and treatment.

1. **Identification and Treatment of Underlying Causes**
    - **Infections**: Antibiotics for infections like urinary tract infections or pneumonia.
    - **Electrolyte Imbalances**: Correcting dehydration, low sodium, or other imbalances.

- **Medications**: Stopping or adjusting drugs that may be contributing to delirium (e.g., sedatives, anticholinergics, opioids, histamine-blocking agents, analgesics, sedative–hypnotics, or cardiovascular drugs).
- **Hypoxia**: Administering oxygen if the patient is experiencing low oxygen levels.
- **Renal or Hepatic Dysfunction**: Treating the underlying kidney or liver issues.

2. **Symptomatic Treatment**

- **Sedation**: In cases of severe agitation or aggression, low doses of antipsychotic medications (e.g., haloperidol) may be used.
- **Benzodiazepines**: Occasionally used for alcohol withdrawal delirium but generally avoided in other cases due to risk of worsening delirium.

3. **Supportive Care**

- **Re-orientation**: Use clocks, calendars, and gentle reminders to help orient the patient to time, place, and person.
- **Hydration and Nutrition**: Ensure the patient is properly hydrated and nourished.
- **Physical Environment**: Provide a calm, quiet, and well-lit environment to reduce confusion.
- **Family Involvement**: Engage family members to provide reassurance and familiarity.

4. **Monitoring and Observation**

- **Frequent Reassessment**: Monitor the patient's mental status regularly and adjust treatment as needed.
- **Prevention of Falls**: Assess the patient's mobility and use safety precautions to prevent falls.

7 Nursing Problems and Interventions of Delirium

Nursing assessment mainly focus on patient's ability to meet basic daily needs, appearance, behavior, duration, and severity of cognitive impairment. Judgment, orientation, memory, affect, and cognition (JOMAC) are key areas of cognitive function to be assessed. After initial assessment and identification of possible aetiological factors, management can be planned. Multidisciplinary and multicomponent interventions aimed at high-risk patients can reduce the chance of development of delirium.

Safe and calm environment

Old age is associated with high risk of falls due to frailty, polypharmacy, and comorbid medical conditions. This can be prevented by using low beds, bed rails, adequate lighting and avoiding physical restraints if possible. Restraints should be used only if patient is a danger to self/others and with proper documentation.

Calm and quiet place helps a patient to reorient to his/her environment. Noise and stimulation should be kept low. A consistent routine should be maintained. Providing comforting and familiar items can aid in reorientation process.

Assistance in meeting basic physiological needs

A nurse should ensure adequate hydration, nutrition, sleep, and bowel-bladder care. Meticulous monitoring for pain, infection, hypoxia or metabolic imbalances are needed, and collaboration with respective physician for proper management is mandatory. Ensuring mobility is another important task for prevention of bed sore.

Stabilization of behavior

Reorientation of the patient frequently can be established by using clock, calendars, and familiar objects in the room. Repeated change of caregiver is not expected. Caregivers should speak clearly and slowly, not confronting the patient for mistakes and avoiding arguments.

Monitor and manage underlying causes

Presence of any potential medication (anticholinergic, opioids) worsens delirium. Nursing staffs should collaborate with physicians to address such medications, infections, electrolyte imbalance, or other causes. Regular monitoring and documentation of vital signs and lab values are other important areas to be taken care of.

Documentation of onset and duration of confusion, behavioral observation, intervention and patient responses, communication with family and physicians helps to monitor the course of the delirium and take necessary steps to prevent deterioration.

8 Medication Management

Work with the healthcare team to review the patient's medication list. Discontinue or adjust any medications that may be contributing to the delirium, such as sedatives or anticholinergic drugs.

If necessary, antipsychotic medications (such as haloperidol) may be prescribed to manage severe agitation or psychosis. Monitor for side effects closely.

Family education and support

Family psychoeducation is an integral part of delirium management, as most patients do not get full recovery during discharge from the hospital. When the family is informed about common precipitating factors, they can prevent the onset or deterioration of the event.

9 Discharge Planning

Ensure that follow-up care is arranged to monitor the patient's cognitive status and prevent recurrence of delirium. Arrange for home care if needed and provide family education on managing confusion at home.

Dementia

Dementia is a major neurocognitive disorder which affects the memory, judgment, and intellect of a person. It usually occurs after 65 years of age; however, though rare, presenile dementia are also found. Worldwide, around 57.6 million population has been affected by Dementia and two-thirds of the cases were reported from low- and middle-income countries. In Bangladesh, the prevalence of dementia is around 8% and females are disproportionately more affected than male. The number is predicted to be doubled in every 20 years posing a major public health concern.

10 Definition of Dementia

Dementia is an acquired global impairment of intellect, memory, and personality, without impairment of consciousness. The core feature that distinguishes dementia from delirium is preservation of consciousness and absence of fluctuating nature. Affected person shows persistent declination of memory, attention, executive function, language, perceptual-motor, or social cognition.

Diagnosis of dementia is based on the clinical history, cognitive assessment by screening tool like Mini-Mental State Examination (MMSE), physical and neurological examination especially for stroke and Parkinsonism and investigations. Investigations are carried out to rule out reversible causes. ICD-11 and DSM-5 define dementia or major neurocognitive disorders with nearly the same criteria, except ICD-11 emphasizes clinical judgment over standardized testing.

11 DSM-5 Diagnostic Criteria for Dementia

DSM-5 uses the term Major and Mild Neurocognitive Disorders. Dementia and Major Neurocognitive Disorders (NCD) are used interchangeably in DSM 5. In broader sense, Major NCDs encompass all the cases with declined function of any single cognitive domain. For diagnosis of dementia, deficits in multiple cognitive domain are required. However, dementia is still used in cases for clinical precision.

In DSM-5, the diagnostic criteria are discussed under major and mild NCD. The specific criteria according to etiological subtypes are discussed separately (e.g., major or mild NCD due to Alzheimer's disease) and beyond the scope of this chapter.

Diagnostic Criteria.

A. Evidence of significant cognitive decline from a previous level of performance in one or more cognitive domains (complex attention, executive function, learning and memory, language, perceptual-motor, or social cognition) based on individual/informant's concern about the impairment and documentation by standardized neuropsychological testing.
B. The cognitive deficits interfere with independence in everyday activities with complex instrumental activities of daily living.
C. The cognitive deficits do not occur exclusively in the context of a delirium.
D. The cognitive deficits are not better explained by another mental disorder (e.g., major depressive disorder, schizophrenia).

Box 1. Types of dementia

Alzheimer's disease
Frontotemporal degeneration
Lewy body disease
Vascular disease
Traumatic brain injury
Substance/medication use
HIV infection
Prion disease
Parkinson's disease
Huntington's disease
Another medical condition
Multiple etiologies
Unspecified etiology

12 Signs/Symptoms of Dementia

Memory impairment in one or more areas is the defining symptoms of Dementia. Other features manifest depending on the subtypes (Box 1, 2). Onset of dementia is gradual and insidious in all types except for vascular dementia due to stroke.

Alzheimer's disease is the most prevalent form of dementia accounting for 50%–60% of all dementias. The early signs are gradual onset of forgetfulness of recent events, word-finding difficulty, loss of orientation to time, place and person, and apathy. In later stage, memory impairment becomes severe and the person needs assistance for daily activities. Impaired judgment, confusion, aphasia (difficulty in expressing language), apraxia (difficulty with motor function, agnosia (difficulty in object recognition) and behavioral and psychological features like suspiciousness, odd behavior, and impaired judgment emerge.

Vascular dementia is the second most common subtype. It emerges after cerebrovascular event and progress in stepwise manner with each recurrent stroke. The general symptoms of dementia are similar to Alzheimer's type.

Frontotemporal type of dementia is associated with atrophy in the frontotemporal regions. The classical clinical feature is changes in behavior and personality with relative preservation of other areas of cognition (e.g., learning, memory, and perceptual-motor function). Social cognition and executive functioning are grossly impaired. Other associated features are disinhibition, apathy, perseveration, stereotypies, and hyperorality.

Dementia with Lewy bodies is caused by the deposition of abnormal proteins made up of alpha-synuclein. Core features are fluctuating cognition, detailed and well-formed visual hallucination, features of Parkinsonism (tremor, rigidity, and bradykinesia) and REM sleep behavior disorder. Patients with Lewy body dementia are prone to develop sensitivity to antipsychotic medication; therefore, those group of drugs should be avoided.

The other dementia subtypes include neurocognitive disorder due to traumatic brain injury, HIV infection, Prion disease, and Huntington disease.

Box 2. Signs/Symptoms of Dementia

- Gradual onset of cognitive decline, with symptoms worsening over time.
- Memory loss, particularly short-term memory.
- Difficulty with language, communication, and understanding.
- Impaired reasoning and judgment, leading to poor decision-making.
- Changes in personality and behavior (e.g., apathy, irritability).
- Difficulty with daily activities (e.g., managing finances, cooking).

13 Risk Factors for Dementia

Risk factors for developing dementia can be broadly classified as modifiable and non-modifiable causes (Table 2).

14 Medical Management of Dementia

Dementia involves a progressive decline in cognitive function, and management focuses on slowing progression, managing symptoms, and improving quality of life. Dementia management usually targeted to the core pathophysiological features and the behavioral and psychological symptoms of dementia. In Alzheimer's disease, brain atrophy is associated with the presence of neurofibrillary tangles and amyloid plaques. There is loss of cholinergic neurons in cerebral cortex and proliferation of astrocytes.

It is recommended that medication for both core features and behavioral problems should be initiated after thorough assessment, addressing the physical and

Table 2 Risk factors of dementia

Non-modifiable risk factors	
Age	Increasing age (>65 years of age)
Family History	Alzheimer's disease, Lewy body dementia
Genetics	*Apo E4,* other genetic polymorphism
Modifiable risk factors	
Cardiovascular Health	Hypertension, dyslipidemia, heart disease
Diabetes	Uncontrolled diabetes
Obesity	Obesity, particularly in midlife
Smoking	Toxins in smoke increase the risk of vascular events
Excessive alcohol consumption	
Physical inactivity	Sedentary life style
Sensory impairment	Untreated hearing and vision impairment
Depression	Depression especially late life depression
Social isolation	Lack of social support and engagement
Traumatic Brain Injury	Head injury especially moderate to severe injuries
Infection	HIV, Syphilis, Lyme disease

environmental precipitating factors and attempting the non-drug measures. Effective evidence-based care in nursing homes significantly reduces the need for psychotropic medications in dementia (Box 3).

Box 3. Medical Management of Dementia

1. **Pharmacological Treatment**
    - **Cholinesterase Inhibitors** (e.g., Donepezil, Rivastigmine, Galantamine): Used for mild to moderate dementia to increase acetylcholine and improve cognitive function.
    - **NMDA Receptor Antagonists** (e.g., Memantine): For moderate-to-severe dementia.
    - **Antidepressants** (e.g., SSRIs like Sertraline, Fluoxetine): For depression or anxiety associated with dementia.
    - **Antipsychotics** (e.g., Risperidone, Olanzapine): Manage behavioral symptoms like aggression and agitation, with caution due to side effects.
    - **Mood Stabilizers** (e.g., Valproic acid, Lithium): Used for mood swings and aggression.
2. **Non-Pharmacological Interventions**
    - **Cognitive Stimulation Therapy**: Activities to encourage memory and cognitive skills.
    - **Cognitive Behavioral Therapy (CBT)**: Addresses anxiety, depression, and coping strategies.

- **Environmental Modifications**: Simplify the environment to reduce confusion (e.g., clear labeling, reducing clutter).
- **Reminiscence Therapy**: Engage in past memories to enhance well-being and memory.

3. **Management of Behavioral Symptoms**

- Cognition-oriented interventions: de-escalation by speaking in calm and quiet voice, maintaining calm gesture, reminiscence therapy, cognitive stimulation therapy.
- Sensory-oriented interventions: Aromatherapy, light therapy, music therapy
- Movement-oriented intervention: Exercise therapy, outdoor activity therapy.

4. **Monitoring and Caregiver Support**

- **Regular Monitoring**: Track cognitive and functional decline with neuropsychiatric assessments.
- **Caregiver Education**: Provide education on dementia progression and coping strategies.
- **Respite Care**: Offer temporary relief for caregivers through professional care.

5. **Treatment of Co-Existing Conditions**

- **Control Comorbidities**: Manage conditions like hypertension, diabetes, and hyperlipidemia to prevent further cognitive decline.

15 Nursing Management of Dementia

Nursing diagnoses of dementia are crucial to avoid misdiagnosis and false labeling, identifying comorbid medical or psychiatric disorder, establishing the need for practical and psychosocial care and the need assessment of the caregivers. A nurse should clinically differentiate between age-related cognitive decline (ARCD), mild cognitive impairment (MCI), and dementia. Mild forgetfulness with no progressive deterioration and no impact on daily functioning is likely due to ARCD. Once the diagnosis of dementia is established, a nurse should assess the person's needs and mental state, including cognitive abilities, behavioral manifestations, and spirituality and sexuality.

Person-centered care

Person-centered care approach will help a nurse to understand the patient beyond diagnosis. Example of person-centered care includes, using patient's first name, acknowledging past roles, adopting a familiar and comfortable routine, addressing the unmet needs etc.

Cognitive stimulation and orientation

Cognitive stimulation and orientation strategies help patient to reorient with the environment. Use of calendar, clock, and verbal reminders are helpful tools. Reminiscing from the past with the help of photo albums and discussion about past memories often rejuvenate the patients.

Managing behavioral and psychological symptoms

Managing behavioral and psychological symptoms (BPSD) is another important domain. Agitation, depression, wandering, aggression, and psychosis (e.g., suspiciousness, hearing or seeing something unseen) are common among the symptoms.

Communication-focused interventions

In dementia, language and processing speed is markedly affected. Using short simple sentences, allowing extra time for the response, avoiding open-ended questions, and giving verbal and nonverbal cues help to improve communication.

Assisting Activities of Daily Living

Assisting Activities of Daily Living (ADLs) is the most important task for nurses. Patients should be encouraged to feed, groom, and dress on their own with minimum assistance, if necessary. An easy-to-follow routine can be applied. Incontinence can be managed by fixing times for toileting and using visual cues to help with toilet identification.

Caregiver education and support

Caregiver education and support by the nursing staff is vital as dementia care extends beyond the patient to the family. Caregivers should be offered psychoeducation about dementia including the nature and progression and the behavioral management strategies. Early identification of caregiver burnout will help to improve their mental health and reduce institutionalization of the patient. Caregivers can be encouraged to take balanced diet, adequate night time sleep, regular physical activity, provide care by rotation, and keep in touch with other caregivers.

Medication management and safety

There is no specific medication to cure neurocognitive disorders. However, patients with dementia may get medication for cognitive enhancement (cholinesterase inhibitors, memantine), BPSD (antidepressant, antipsychotics), or other comorbid medical conditions. Special attention is needed to address the efficacy of existing medication and adverse effects of any newly added or dose increased medication. Fall can be prevented by using bed/chair alarms, adequate lighting, and removal of hazards. Hydration, nutrition, and personal hygiene should be properly maintained. End-of-life care preferences can be discussed as a part of advanced care planning.

Promoting quality of life requires the provision of opportunities for engagement in meaningful activities, including hobbies and passions to support psychological well-being. Maintaining regular social interaction is essential to prevent social isolation; this may be facilitated through scheduled visits, community involvement, and other forms of interpersonal contact. Advance care planning encompasses early discussion of anticipated future needs, including preferences for end-of-life care and relevant legal considerations. In the later stages of illness, emphasis should be placed on palliative interventions aimed at maintaining dignity, alleviating discomfort, and supporting the individual's overall comfort. Continuous monitoring and systematic documentation are critical components of care, involving regular reassessment to identify changes in condition and vigilant observation for any deterioration that may necessitate timely medical intervention.

Life expectancy in Bangladesh has been increased to 73–75 years. This in turn contributes to the increased dementia burden. With limited skilled manpower and inadequate infrastructures, dementia will pose a major public health concern. A holistic, evidence-based, comprehensive nursing care can ensure better psychosocial outcome for both the patient with dementia and the caregivers.

Take Home Message

- Delirium and dementia are the most common neurocognitive disorder in late age. Core feature of delirium is altered level of consciousness whereas core feature of dementia is progressive loss of memory.
- Delirium is multifactorial in nature. Dementia is caused by multiple etiologies. The common risk factors are old age, preexisting cognitive dysfunction, and medical comorbidities.
- Early identification of precipitating factor and timely intervention can reverse or halt progression of delirium.
- In dementia, symptomatic management, management of medical comorbidities, and management of behavioral and psychological symptoms are areas to be focused.
- Nursing interventions include thorough assessment, assessment of needs, helping with ADLs, and support for the caregivers.
- Holistic, evidence-based, comprehensive nursing care ensures the better patient outcome in delirium and dementia.

Sample Short Answer Questions

1. Define delirium and/or dementia.
2. Mention common causes/etiology/risk factors of delirium/dementia.
3. Mention the signs and symptoms of delirium/dementia.

Sample Essay Questions

1. Explain the medical management of delirium/dementia.

2. As a psychiatric nurse, how will you manage a case of delirium/dementia in the ward?

Sample Multiple Choice Questions (MCQ) and Best Answer Question

Signs/symptoms of dementia involve-			Which symptom is most commonly associated with delirium?		
T	a)	Dementia causes memory loss		a)	Slow cognitive decline
F	b)	Dementia symptoms don't stay stable	✓	b)	Rapid confusion
T	c)	Dementia affects cognitive function		c)	Consistent memory
F	d)	Dementia causes rapid onset confusion		d)	Impaired judgment
T	e)	Dementia involves gradual decline over time			

Suggested Reading

Arafat, S. M. Y., Mazumder, A. H. (2025). Geriatric psychiatry in Bangladesh: Current status and Ways Ahead. In N. Kar, S. K. Kar, & S. M. Y. Arafat (Eds.), Geriatric psychiatry in South Asia. South Asian perspectives in mental health and psychology. Springer. https://doi.org/10.1007/978-981-96-7469-5_2

Boland, R. J., Verduin, M. L., & Ruiz, P. (2022). Kaplan & Sadock's synopsis of psychiatry (12th ed.). Wolters Kluwer.

Fossey, J., Ballard, C., Juszczak, E., James, I., Alder, N., Jacoby, R., & Howard, R. (2006). Effect of enhanced psychosocial care on antipsychotic use in nursing home residents with severe dementia: Cluster randomised trial. *BMJ (Clinical research ed.), 332*(7544), 756–761. https://doi.org/10.1136/bmj.38782.575868.7C

Harrison, P. J., Cowen, P. J., Burns, T., & Fazel, M. (2018). *Shorter Oxford textbook of psychiatry* (7th ed.).

Hategan, A., Bourgeois, J. A., Cheng, T., & Young, J. S. (2018). *Geriatric psychiatry study guide: Mastering the competencies* (1st ed.). Springer. https://doi.org/10.1007/978-3-319-77128-1

Inouye, S. K., Westendrop, R. G. J., & Saczynski, J. S. (2014). Delirium in elderly people. *Lancet, 383*(9920), 911–922.

Kim, S. K., & Park, M. (2017). Effectiveness of person-centered care on people with dementia: A systematic review and meta-analysis. *Clinical interventions in aging, 12*, 381–397. https://doi.org/10.2147/CIA.S117637

Meagher, D. J., Moran, M., Raju, B., Gibbons, D., Donnelly, S., Saunders, J., & Trzepacz, P. T. (2007). Phenomenology of delirium. Assessment of 100 adult cases using standardised measures. *The British Journal of Psychiatry: The Journal of Mental Science, 190*, 135–141. https://doi.org/10.1192/bjp.bp.106.023911

Naheed, A., Hakim, M., Islam, M. S., Islam, M. B., Tang, E. Y. H., Prodhan, A. A., Amin, M. R., Stephan, B. C. M., & Mohammad, Q. D. (2023). Prevalence of dementia among older age people and variation across different sociodemographic characteristics: A cross-sectional study in Bangladesh. *The Lancet regional health. Southeast Asia, 17*, Article 100257. https://doi.org/10.1016/j.lansea.2023.100257

Needham, J. (2006). *Alzheimer's disease. CME resource: Continuing education for Florida nurses* (pp. 69–122). Continuing Medical Education, Inc.

Shives, L. R. (2011). *Basic concepts of psychiatric–Mental health nursing.* (8th ed.). Lippincott Williams & Wilkins.

Taylor, D., Barnes, T. R. E., & Young, A. H. (2025). *The Maudsley prescribing guidelines in psychiatry* (15th ed.). Wiley-Blackwell.

Vasilevskis, E. E., Han, J. H., Hughes, C. G., & Ely, E. W. (2012). Epidemiology and risk factors for delirium across hospital settings. *Best Practice & research. Clinical Anaesthesiology, 26*(3), 277–287. https://doi.org/10.1016/j.bpa.2012.07.003

Wang, G., Albayrak, A., & van der Cammen, T. J. M. (2019). A systematic review of non-pharmacological interventions for BPSD in nursing home residents with dementia: From a perspective of ergonomics. *International Psychogeriatrics, 31*(8), 1137–1149. https://doi.org/10.1017/S1041610218001679

Chapter 11
Care of Clients with Substance Use Disorders and Substance-Related Disorders

Hasina Akter and S. M. Yasir Arafat

Abstract Substance abuse disorders are major health and social problems in Bangladesh. They involve harmful use of substances such as yaba, heroin, phensedyl, and cannabis. This chapter highlights diagnostic criteria as per international guidelines, drug abuse, tolerance, and withdrawal. Risk factors include peer influence, family dysfunction, poverty, and easy access to drugs. Management includes detoxification, pharmacotherapy, counseling, and rehabilitation. Nurses address problems like risk of injury, malnutrition, and altered behavior through safety measures, education, and support. Prevention relies on awareness programs, family support, school education, and strong community-based strategies.

Keywords Substance abuse disorders · Risk factors · DSM-5 diagnostic criteria · Medical and nursing management · Prevention strategies

The World Health Organization (WHO) defines substance use disorders as the harmful or hazardous use of psychoactive substances (like alcohol and illicit drugs) that leads to clinically significant damage to a person's physical or mental health, or results in behaviors that harm others. This includes patterns of use that result in physical dependence (characterized by tolerance and withdrawal symptoms) and an impaired control over substance use, with a strong desire or craving to use the substance. The WHO classifies these disorders, often referred to as addiction, as health conditions that should be addressed within the healthcare system, rather than through criminal justice.

The WHO defines drug abuse as the harmful or hazardous use of psychoactive substances. This includes alcohol and both illicit and prescription drugs, which cause damage to physical or mental health. The WHO emphasizes that this pattern of

H. Akter
Department of Graduate Nursing, Bangladesh Medical University, Dhaka, Bangladesh

S. M. Y. Arafat (✉)
Department of Psychiatry, Bangladesh Specialized Hospital, Dhaka, Bangladesh
e-mail: arafatdmc62@gmail.com

S. M. Y. Arafat and H. Akter (eds.), *Psychiatric Nursing in Bangladesh*, Mental Health Systems and Policy in Low- and Middle-Income Countries,
https://doi.org/10.1007/978-981-95-8501-4_11

use can lead to drug use disorders, which are characterized by a strong desire to consume the substance, difficulty controlling use, and persistent use despite harmful consequences.

Drug dependence, as defined by WHO, is a condition characterized by the compulsive use of a psychoactive substance, with a strong desire to take the substance regularly. This includes a variety of physiological and behavioral symptoms, including tolerance, withdrawal symptoms, and compulsive drug-seeking behavior. Drug dependence leads to physical or psychological dependence, and it interferes with the person's social, occupational, and recreational functioning.

Drug tolerance refers to the process by which the body becomes accustomed to the effects of a drug, leading to a diminished response to the same dose. As tolerance develops, an individual may require larger doses of the substance to achieve the same effects that were previously attained with smaller doses. Tolerance is a key feature of substance dependence and is part of the adaptive physiological changes that occur with prolonged use.

Withdrawal state, according to WHO, refers to a set of physical and mental symptoms that occur when a person who is dependent on a substance reduces or ceases its use. These symptoms can range from mild to severe, depending on the drug involved and the individual's level of dependence. Symptoms of withdrawal may include anxiety, sweating, nausea, headaches, tremors, and in severe cases, seizures or delirium. WHO recognizes withdrawal as a key feature of substance dependence and an indicator of the need for interventions.

1 Epidemiology of Substance Abuse in Bangladesh

In Bangladesh, substance abuse has become a significant public health concern, with epidemiological data indicating a growing burden, particularly among youth. National estimates from the National Institute of Mental Health (NIMH) and the United Nations Office on Drugs and Crime (UNODC) suggest that approximately 3.6 million people in the country use drugs. A household survey conducted in 2017–2018 reported a prevalence of 2–3% among children and adolescents, highlighting early initiation of substance use. Commonly abused substances include cannabis, heroin, phensedyl (codeine cough syrup), and yaba, which has emerged as the most frequently used stimulant (Box 1). Studies among school and university students further indicate vulnerability among young populations, with lifetime prevalence rates for tobacco, alcohol, and illicit drugs ranging from 10 to 15% in some groups. Hospital- and clinic-based studies corroborate the rising dominance of yaba, followed by heroin, cannabis, and phensedyl in treatment settings. A narrative review of 15 studies reported that the majority of substance users are male (94.17%), predominantly young adults under 30 years, and mostly unmarried (62.90%), with a high proportion from urban areas (94.17%). Heroin, followed by yaba and cannabis, was the most commonly reported substance of first use, and many individuals engage in poly-substance use. Routes of administration are mainly oral or inhalation, with injection less frequent. Another study highlighted the co-existence of substance use and mental health conditions, reporting that in a sample of 115 individuals, over 90% were male, with a mean age of 24.6 years, and about half were in the 21–30 year age group. Nicotine use was almost universal (94.8%), followed by cannabinoids (56.5%) and opiates (38.3%), while psychiatric comorbidities were present in 29.6% of participants and physical comorbidities in approximately one-third. Overall, these findings indicate that substance abuse in Bangladesh typically begins in young adulthood, is heavily male-dominated, more prevalent in urban settings, frequently involves multiple substances, and often co-exists with mental health problems. Despite these insights, there remains a lack of large-scale nationwide studies using formal diagnostic criteria to determine the full prevalence of substance use disorder in the general population.

Box 1: Common Types of Substances Used in Bangladesh

- **Tobacco (Cigarettes, Bidis, Smokeless Tobacco)**

  Tobacco use is widespread in Bangladesh, with cigarettes and bidis (a traditional hand-rolled cigarette) being commonly used. Smokeless tobacco is also popular in the form of zarda or tobacco paste.

- **Cannabis (Marijuana or Ganja)**

  Cannabis is illegally cultivated and widely used in various regions. The substance is often used recreationally.

- **Heroin and Other Opiates**

  Heroin use is prevalent, especially in urban areas. It is typically injected or smoked, and its abuse has been increasing in recent years.

- **Pharmaceutical Drugs**

  Benzodiazepines and other prescription medications, often used for anxiety or sleep disorders, are abused by many individuals in Bangladesh. Sedatives like clonazepam, diazepam, or alprazolam are abused, especially in urban populations. Painkillers such as codeine and tramadol are also commonly misused, often in combination with other substances.

- **Inhalants (E.g., Glue, Paint Thinner, and Other Volatile Substances)**

  Inhalants are particularly abused by adolescents and individuals living in poverty-stricken areas. They are easily accessible and can produce short-term euphoric effects.

- **Ecstasy (MDMA) and Other Party Drugs**

Although not as common as other drugs, the use of ecstasy and other club drugs like LSD is reported, particularly in some urban areas, including during social gatherings or parties.

- **Alcohol**

  Alcohol consumption is prevalent in certain social groups, although cultural and religious factors may influence its usage. It's one of the most commonly abused substances in Bangladesh.

2 Etiology/Risk Factors of Substance Use Disorders

a) **Genetic Factors**

- Family history of substance abuse or addiction increases the risk.
- Genetic predisposition can influence how the brain responds to substances, making some more susceptible.

b) **Psychological Factors**

- Mental health conditions may lead to self-medication with substances.
- Stress, trauma, and childhood abuse can increase the risk.

c) **Environmental Factors**

- Peer pressure or social groups that encourage substance use, especially during adolescence, increase risk.
- Dysfunctional family dynamics or exposure to substance use within the household can normalize abuse.
- Cultural and societal attitudes toward substances influence behavior.

d) **Availability and Accessibility of Substances**

- Easy access to drugs, or prescriptions, increases misuse.
- Lower socio-economic status may heighten exposure to substance use as a coping mechanism.

e) **Neurological and Biological Factors**

- Substance use alters brain chemistry, impacting reward, decision-making, and self-control.
- Neurotransmitter imbalances (e.g., dopamine or serotonin dysfunction) contribute to cravings and dependence.

f) **Environmental and Social Stressors**

- Stressors like unemployment, poverty, or social isolation can increase vulnerability to substance abuse.

g) **Co-occurring Disorders**

- Individuals with mental health disorders like anxiety or depression are at higher risk of substance misuse due to self-medication.

h) **Early Age of Initiation**

- Early substance use during adolescence increases the likelihood of developing a substance use disorder.

i) **Trauma and Life Experiences**

- Childhood trauma (e.g., abuse, violence) or life transitions (e.g., divorce, loss) can increase the risk of substance abuse.

j) **Personality Traits and Coping Mechanisms**

- Impulsivity, poor coping skills, and lack of emotional regulation increase the likelihood of turning to substances to manage difficult emotions.

3 Signs/Symptoms of Substance Abuse Disorders

The signs and symptoms of substance abuse disorders can vary depending on the substance being abused, but some common signs and symptoms include:

A) **Physical Symptoms**

a) **Changes in appearance**

- Sudden weight loss or gain.
- Poor personal hygiene.
- Red or bloodshot eyes.
- Dilated or constricted pupils.
- Unexplained tremors or shakiness.
- Nosebleeds (in case of snorting drugs).

b) **Health Issues**

- Chronic cough or shortness of breath (especially with smoking or inhalant abuse).
- Frequent infections or illnesses (due to weakened immune system).
- Liver damage, liver enlargement, or jaundice (in alcohol or drug abuse).
- Nausea, vomiting, or abdominal pain.
- Poor coordination and balance.

a) **Sleep Disturbance**

- Insomnia or excessive drowsiness.

B) **Behavioral Symptoms**

a) **Changes in Social Behavior**

- Social isolation or withdrawal from family and friends.
- Engaging in risky or dangerous behaviors (e.g., driving under the influence).
- Neglecting responsibilities at home, work, or school.

b) **Secretive or Suspicious Behavior**

- Lying about activities or whereabouts.
- Hiding substances or paraphernalia.
- Frequently borrowing money or stealing.

c) **Frequent Mood Swings**

- Extreme irritability, agitation, or euphoria.
- Sudden bursts of anger or aggression.
- Depression or withdrawal.

d) **Poor Judgment and Decision-Making**

- Engaging in reckless activities or behaviors.
- Lack of concern for personal safety or well-being.

e) **Inability to Stop or Control Substance Use**

- Frequent unsuccessful attempts to cut down or quit using the substance.
- Craving or intense urge to use the substance.

C) **Psychological Symptoms**

a) **Changes in Mental State**

- Anxiety, depression, or paranoia.
- Hallucinations, delusions, or confusion (especially with heavy drug use).
- Lack of motivation (apathy).

b) **Cognitive Impairment**

- Memory problems or difficulty concentrating.
- Impaired judgment and problem-solving skills.

D) **Tolerance and Withdrawal Symptoms**

a) **Tolerance**

- Needing increasing amounts of the substance to achieve the same effect.

b) **Withdrawal Symptoms**

- Sweating, shaking, or nausea when not using the substance.
- Difficulty sleeping or intense cravings.
- Muscle pain, tremors, or seizures (for some substances).

4 Diagnostic Criteria for Substance Use Disorder

The *Diagnostic and Statistical Manual of Mental Disorders*, 5th Edition (DSM-5) defines Substance Use Disorder (SUD) as a condition involving the problematic use of alcohol, drugs, or other substances that leads to significant impairment or distress. The criteria for diagnosing substance use disorder require evidence of at least two of the following symptoms occurring within a 12-month period:

- Substance is often taken in larger amounts or over a longer period than was intended.
- There is a persistent desire or unsuccessful efforts to cut down or control substance use.
- A great deal of time is spent in activities to obtain, use, or recover from the effects of the substance.
- Craving, or a strong desire or urge to use the substance.
- Recurrent substance use resulting in a failure to fulfill major role obligations at work, school, or home.
- Continued substance use despite having persistent or recurrent social or interpersonal problems caused or worsened by the effects of the substance.
- Important social, occupational, or recreational activities are given up or reduced because of substance use.
- Recurrent substance use in situations in which it is physically hazardous.
- Substance use is continued despite knowing of a persistent or recurrent physical or psychological problem likely to have been caused or worsened by the substance.
- Tolerance (e.g., needing more of the substance to achieve the desired effect or diminished effect with continued use of the same amount).
- Withdrawal (e.g., experiencing withdrawal symptoms when the substance use is reduced or discontinued).

Impaired control 4 items (1–4), social problem 3 items (5–7), risky behavior 2 items (8–9), dependence 2 items (10,11).

5 Medical Management of Substance Use Disorders

The treatment for substance use disorders typically involves a combination of detoxification, medication, psychotherapy, and supportive care. The specific approach depends on the substance involved and the severity of the disorder.

a) **Detoxification**

   - The initial phase, where the substance is cleared from the body, typically in a medical setting to manage withdrawal symptoms and ensure safety.

- For alcohol or sedative withdrawal, benzodiazepines may be used.

b) **Pharmacological Treatment**

- **Opioid Use Disorder**: Methadone, buprenorphine, or naltrexone.
- **Alcohol Use Disorder**: Disulfiram, acamprosate, or naltrexone.
- **Nicotine Dependence**: Nicotine replacement therapies, varenicline, or bupropion.
- **Stimulant Use Disorder**: Behavioral treatments are emphasized as there are no FDA-approved medications.

c) **Psychotherapy**

- **Cognitive-Behavioral Therapy (CBT)**: Helps identify and change behaviors related to substance use.
- **Motivational Interviewing (MI)**: Increases motivation to change substance use.
- **Contingency Management**: Rewards for maintaining abstinence.
- **12-Step Programs**: Support groups like Alcoholics Anonymous (AA) and Narcotics Anonymous (NA).

d) **Relapse Prevention**

- Teaching coping skills to handle triggers and high-risk situations.
- Ongoing support groups and counseling sessions for long-term management.

e) **Family and Social Support**

- Family therapy to address dynamics that contribute to addiction.
- Support from family and friends is essential for recovery.

f) **Inpatient vs. Outpatient Care**

- **Inpatient Care**: For severe addiction or complex medical conditions requiring intensive supervision.
- **Outpatient Care**: Suitable for milder disorders or post-inpatient treatment.

g) **Aftercare**

- Ongoing therapy, participation in support groups, and continued support from healthcare providers for long-term recovery and relapse prevention.

6 Nursing Management of Substance Use Disorders

As a psychiatric nurse, managing a case of substance abuse disorder involves providing comprehensive care that addresses both the physical and psychological aspects of the disorder (Table 1). The preventive measures have been mentioned in Table 2.

Table 1 Nursing care plan table for clients with substance-related disorders

Assessment	Nursing diagnosis	Goals/Planning	Nursing interventions	Evaluation
• History of substance use (type, frequency, amount) • Physical signs of withdrawal or intoxication • Client reports craving and inability to control use—possible legal or social problems related to substance use	1. Risk for Injury related to impaired judgment and withdrawal symptoms	Client will remain free from injury during withdrawal and treatment	• Monitor vital signs and withdrawal symptoms closely • Ensure a safe environment to prevent falls or accidents • Administer prescribed medications to manage withdrawal • Educate client about risks of substance use	Client remains free from injuries, and withdrawal is safely managed
• Ineffective coping mechanisms • Client expresses feelings of guilt, shame, or denial • Lack of social support or unstable family relationships	2. Ineffective Coping related to substance dependence and psychosocial stressors	Client will demonstrate adaptive coping skills and express feelings appropriately	• Encourage verbalization of feelings and thoughts • Teach stress management and relaxation techniques • Refer to counseling or support groups (e.g., AA, NA) • Involve family in therapy sessions if appropriate	Client uses positive coping strategies and participates in therapy/support groups

(continued)

Table 1 (continued)

Assessment	Nursing diagnosis	Goals/Planning	Nursing interventions	Evaluation
• Nutritional deficiencies and poor self-care • Sleep disturbances and fatigue • Risk for infection due to weakened immunity	3. Imbalanced Nutrition: Less Than Body Requirements related to poor intake and substance effects	Client will maintain adequate nutrition and hydration	• Assess nutritional status and offer balanced meals/snacks • Encourage fluid intake • Monitor weight and lab values • Collaborate with dietitian for specialized diet plans	Client maintains or improves nutritional status and hydration
• Knowledge deficit about effects of substance abuse and treatment options	4. Deficient Knowledge related to lack of information about substance abuse and recovery	Client will verbalize understanding of substance abuse effects and treatment plan	• Provide information about the substance, its effects, and risks • Educate about treatment options and relapse prevention • Use simple language and written materials • Reinforce teaching regularly	Client demonstrates understanding and engages in treatment plan
• Social isolation and withdrawal from activities	5. Social Isolation related to substance abuse and its psychosocial effects	Client will participate in social and recreational activities	• Encourage involvement in support groups • Facilitate family involvement and social support • Promote engagement in meaningful activities	Client increases social interactions and demonstrates improved mood

Table 2 Prevention of substance abuse

Strategy	Description
Education and Awareness	• Run public awareness campaigns • Implement school programs to teach risks and coping skills
Early Intervention	• Screen at-risk individuals early • Provide counseling and early support services
Family Support and Education	• Educate parents on signs of substance abuse • Strengthen family communication and bonding
Healthy Lifestyles & Coping	• Promote physical health, mental wellness, and stress management • Train on resilience skills
Reducing Availability & Access	• Enforce laws on age restrictions • Monitor prescription drug distribution
Peer Education & Support	• Train peer educators to guide and support others in prevention efforts
Community & Social Support	• Build youth engagement programs • Provide support for vulnerable and marginalized groups
Legal and Policy Interventions	• Enact and enforce substance control laws • Implement community-level law enforcement
Treatment & Rehabilitation	• Ensure access to addiction treatment and rehabilitation services
Addressing Mental Health	• Provide integrated mental health and addiction care to reduce self-medication risk

a) **Assessment and Evaluation**:

- **Initial Assessment**: Understand substance use history, withdrawal symptoms, and co-occurring conditions.
- **Mental State Examination**: Evaluate mood, cognition, and behavior for signs of psychosis or anxiety.

b) **Provide Physical Care**:

- **Withdrawal Management**: Monitor and manage withdrawal symptoms, administer medications (e.g., benzodiazepines), and ensure hydration and nutrition.
- **Medical Management**: Manage co-occurring conditions (e.g., anxiety, depression) and monitor medication side effects.

c) **Psychological Support and Counseling**:

- **Therapeutic Communication**: Build trust through active listening and empathetic communication.
- **Motivational Interviewing**: Explore ambivalence and enhance motivation for change.
- **Psychoeducation**: Educate on substance abuse effects and relapse prevention.

d) **Address Co-occurring Mental Health Conditions**:

- **Dual Diagnosis Care**: Collaborate with mental health professionals to treat both substance use and mental health disorders.

e) **Family Involvement**:

- **Support for Families**: Educate and involve family in the treatment process, and encourage family therapy.

f) **Social and Community Support**:

- **Referral to Support Groups**: Refer to Alcoholics Anonymous (AA), Narcotics Anonymous (NA), or other peer groups.
- **Developing a Support Network**: Assist with building a strong support system, including social workers and community resources.

g) **Relapse Prevention and Aftercare**:

- **Create a Relapse Prevention Plan**: Identify triggers and coping strategies.
- **Long-Term Care Planning**: Encourage ongoing therapy and participation in support groups.

h) **Maintain a Safe and Supportive Environment**:

- **Create a Therapeutic Environment**: Ensure a substance-free and supportive setting.
- **Manage Challenging Behaviors**: Address aggression and impulsivity professionally.

i) **Documentation and Reporting**:

- **Document Observations**: Accurately record assessments, interventions, and progress while maintaining confidentiality (Table 1).

Take Home Message

- Substance abuse disorders involve harmful use, tolerance, and withdrawal.
- Commonly abused substances in Bangladesh include tobacco, cannabis, yaba, heroin, alcohol, and phensedyl.
- Risk factors include peer influence, poverty, family dysfunction, and easy drug access.
- Major symptoms are craving, loss of control, neglect of duties, tolerance, and withdrawal.
- DSM-5 diagnosis is based on impaired control, social impairment, risky use, and pharmacological criteria.
- Management requires detoxification, pharmacotherapy, counseling, and rehabilitation.

- Nurses address injury risk, malnutrition, and altered behavior through safety, education, and support.
- Prevention depends on awareness, family involvement, school education, and community strategies.

Sample Multiple Choice (MCQ) and Sample Best Answer Questions

Etiology of Substance Abuse Disorders involves-			Which is a sign of substance abuse?		
T	a)	Genetics affect substance abuse risk		a)	Consistent mood
F	b)	Environment alone causes substance abuse	✓	b)	Withdrawal symptoms
T	c)	Mental health issues may lead to substance abuse		c)	Increased social activity
F	d)	Social status doesn't influence substance abuse		d)	Improved relationships
T	e)	Family history increases substance abuse risk			

Suggested Reading

Kamal, M., Huq, N., Mali, B., Akter, H., & Arafat, S. M. Y. (2018). Epidemiology of substance abuse in Bangladesh: A narrative review. *Journal of Mental Disorders and Treatment, 4*, 165. https://doi.org/10.4172/2471-271X.1000165

Maruf, M. M., Chowdhury, A., Islam, M. R. (2024). Substance use and mental health conditions: Co-existence of dual problems in Bangladesh. In S. M. Y.Arafat (Eds.), *Mental health in Bangladesh.* Springer. https://doi.org/10.1007/978-981-97-0610-5_7

National Institute of Mental Health (NIMH). (2018). *Household survey on substance use among children and adolescents in Bangladesh.* NIMH.

United Nations Office on Drugs and Crime (UNODC). (2021). *Country report on drug use in Bangladesh.* UNODC.

Chapter 12
Care of Clients with Sexual Disorders

Bithika Mali and S. M. Yasir Arafat

Abstract Sexual disorders are prevalent yet often under-recognized conditions that significantly impact psychological well-being, interpersonal relationships, and overall quality of life. This chapter aims to equip nursing students with essential knowledge and practical skills to assess, manage, and support individuals affected by sexual disorders, thereby contributing to holistic sexual health promotion and patient-centered care. It provides a comprehensive overview of sexual disorders with special emphasis on definitions, classifications, risk factors, clinical features, diagnostic criteria, and management strategies. It highlights the multifactorial etiology of sexual dysfunctions, including biological, psychological, relational, sociocultural, and lifestyle components. Current evidence-based approaches in medical management, such as pharmacological therapy, psychotherapy, behavioral interventions, and hormonal treatment, are discussed. The role of nurses is explored in depth, focusing on assessment, therapeutic communication, patient education, supportive interventions, and collaborative care. Preventive measures across primary, secondary, and tertiary levels are also presented.

Keywords Sexual disorders · ICD-11 · DSM-5 · Sexual dysfunction · Nursing management · Sexual health

1 Introduction

Sexual health is a vital component of overall human well-being and quality of life. The World Health Organization (WHO) defines sexual health as a state of physical, emotional, mental, and social well-being related to sexuality, not merely the absence of disease or dysfunction. However, many individuals experience difficulties in sexual

B. Mali
Department of Graduate Nursing, Bangladesh Medical University, Dhaka, Bangladesh

S. M. Y. Arafat (✉)
Department of Psychiatry, Bangladesh Specialized Hospital, Dhaka, Bangladesh
e-mail: arafatdmc62@gmail.com

S. M. Y. Arafat and H. Akter (eds.), *Psychiatric Nursing in Bangladesh*, Mental Health Systems and Policy in Low- and Middle-Income Countries,
https://doi.org/10.1007/978-981-95-8501-4_12

functioning at some point in life, which may lead to distress, relationship problems, and reduced life satisfaction.

Sexual disorders, also known as sexual dysfunctions, encompass a wide range of conditions that affect sexual desire, arousal, orgasm, or cause pain during sexual activity. These disorders can occur in both men and women and may stem from physiological, psychological, or sociocultural factors. Common examples include erectile dysfunction, premature ejaculation, female arousal disorder, and genito-pelvic pain disorders.

For nursing professionals, understanding sexual disorders is crucial because sexuality is an integral part of holistic patient care. Nurses often serve as the first point of contact for patients experiencing such problems. Hence, they must possess the knowledge, sensitivity, and communication skills required to assess, manage, and counsel individuals with sexual health concerns in a non-judgmental and empathetic manner.

2 Sexual Disorders

Sexual disorders refer to a group of conditions characterized by disturbances in a person's ability to respond sexually or to experience sexual pleasure. These disturbances may involve sexual desire, arousal, orgasm, or pain associated with sexual activity. Sexual disorders are **persistent or recurrent disturbances** in sexual desire, arousal, orgasm, or pain during sexual activity that cause **marked distress or interpersonal difficulty**. According to the *International Classification of Diseases* 11th Revision (ICD-11) and *Diagnostic and Statistical Manual of Mental Disorders* (DSM-5), sexual disorders are clinically significant disturbances that cause distress or interpersonal difficulties and are not better explained by medical, psychiatric, or substance-related causes.

3 Common Types of Sexual Disorders According to ICD-11

The **ICD-11** categorizes sexual disorders into several groups, based on which aspect of sexual functioning is affected. The DSM-5 classification is mentioned in Table 1.

1. **Disorders of Sexual Desire and Arousal**
    - **Hypoactive Sexual Desire Disorder (HSDD):** Persistent or recurrent deficiency of sexual thoughts or desire for sexual activity.
    - **Sexual Aversion Disorder:** Extreme aversion to sexual contact or activity.
    - **Erectile Dysfunction (ED):** Inability to achieve or maintain an erection sufficient for satisfactory sexual performance.
    - **Female Sexual Interest/Arousal Disorder:** Lack of or reduced sexual interest, thoughts, or pleasure during sexual activity.

Table 1 Sexual disorders according to DSM-5

Disorder	Primary feature
Female Sexual Interest/Arousal Disorder	Lack of sexual interest, absent/reduced erotic thoughts
Male Hypoactive Sexual Desire Disorder	Persistent low desire
Erectile Disorder	Difficulty obtaining/maintaining erection
Premature Ejaculation	Occurs within 1 min of penetration
Genito-Pelvic Pain/Penetration Disorder	Pain, fear, tensing of pelvic muscles

2. **Orgasmic Disorders**
   - **Delayed Ejaculation:** Marked delay or absence of ejaculation during sexual activity.
   - **Premature (Early) Ejaculation:** Ejaculation that occurs sooner than desired, causing distress.
   - **Female Orgasmic Disorder:** Delay or absence of orgasm following normal sexual arousal.
3. **Sexual Pain Disorders**
   - **Dyspareunia:** Persistent or recurrent pain during sexual intercourse.
   - **Vaginismus:** Involuntary contraction of vaginal muscles, making penetration painful or impossible.
   - **Genito-Pelvic Pain/Penetration Disorder:** Combined pain, fear, or tightening of pelvic muscles during penetration.
4. **Paraphilic Disorders**
   - **Exhibitionistic Disorder:** Sexual arousal from exposing genitals to unsuspecting individuals.
   - **Voyeuristic Disorder:** Sexual arousal from observing unsuspecting people naked or engaging in sexual activity.
   - **Frotteuristic Disorder:** Touching or rubbing against non-consenting individuals.
   - **Pedophilic Disorder:** Sexual attraction to prepubescent children.
   - **Sexual Sadism/Masochism:** Deriving sexual pleasure from inflicting or receiving pain.
5. **Gender Incongruence**
   - **Gender Incongruence of Adolescence or Adulthood:** A marked incongruence between experienced gender and assigned sex.
   - **Gender Incongruence of Childhood:** Persistent desire to be of another gender and discomfort with assigned sex.

4 Risk Factors for Sexual Disorders

The risk factors are mentioned in Box 1.

Box 1. Risk Factors for Sexual Disorders

1. **Biological Factors**
   - Hormonal imbalances (low testosterone, estrogen deficiency)
   - Chronic diseases (diabetes, hypertension, cardiovascular disease)
   - Neurological disorders (spinal cord injury, multiple sclerosis)
   - Side effects of certain medications (antidepressants, antihypertensives)
   - Aging
2. **Psychological Factors**
   - Anxiety and depression
   - Stress and fatigue
   - Relationship conflicts
   - Past sexual trauma or abuse
   - Negative body image or low self-esteem
3. **Social and Cultural Factors**
   - Cultural taboos or religious restrictions
   - Lack of sexual education
   - Marital or communication problems
   - Substance abuse (alcohol, drugs)
4. **Relationship Factors**
   - Marital conflict
   - Lack of intimacy or trust
   - Poor communication
5. **Sociocultural Factors**
   - Restrictions around sexuality
   - Restrictive religious beliefs
   - Misinformation or lack of sexual education
6. **Lifestyle Factors**
   - Alcohol or substance use
   - Smoking
   - Sedentary lifestyle

5 Signs and Symptoms of Sexual Disorders

Sexual disorders manifest through a group of self-reported symptoms (subjective experiences) and observable signs (objective findings) that cause significant distress to the individual. The clinical presentation is typically organized according to the phase of the sexual response cycle that is affected.

1. **Desire (Interest/Arousal) Disorders**
   - **Markedly reduced or absent sexual interest or fantasies:** The individual reports a persistent lack of motivation for sexual activity and a deficiency in spontaneous erotic thoughts.
   - **Absence of responsive desire:** Failure to become aroused in the presence of sexual stimuli, even if spontaneous desire is low.
   - **Aversion to sexual contact:** Active avoidance of genital contact with a partner, which may be accompanied by anxiety, fear, or disgust.
2. **Arousal Disorders**
   - **In women:** Difficulty attaining or maintaining adequate genital lubrication and vulvovaginal swelling during sexual activity, often leading to discomfort or pain.
   - **In men:** Persistent or recurrent inability to achieve or maintain an erection sufficient for sexual performance.
   - **Reduced subjective arousal:** A reported disconnect between physical genital response and the feeling of mental or psychological excitement.
3. **Orgasm Disorders**
   - **Delayed Ejaculation (in men):** A marked delay in, marked infrequency of, or absence of ejaculation despite adequate stimulation.
   - **Premature (Early) Ejaculation (in men):** A pattern of ejaculation occurring within approximately one minute of vaginal penetration and before it is personally desired.
   - **Female Orgasmic Disorder:** A persistent delay in, marked infrequency of, or absence of orgasm, or a markedly reduced intensity of orgasmic sensations.
   - **Anorgasmia:** The general term for the inability to achieve orgasm after sufficient stimulation.
4. **Sexual Pain Disorders**
   - **Dyspareunia:** Persistent or recurrent genital pain experienced during or after sexual intercourse, reported by both men and women.
   - **Vaginismus:** A history of difficulty with vaginal penetration during intercourse or gynecological examination, often due to involuntary spasms of the pelvic floor muscles. This may be accompanied by fear and anticipation of pain.

- **Non-Coital Sexual Pain:** Genital pain induced by non-penetrative sexual stimulation.

5. **Associated Psychological and Relational Features**

Beyond the specific sexual symptoms, individuals often present with co-occurring psychological and interpersonal signs, including:

- **Clinically significant distress:** Feelings of frustration, shame, guilt, anxiety, embarrassment, or low self-esteem directly related to the sexual problem.
- **Depression and anxiety:** These are common comorbidities that can be either a cause or a consequence of the sexual disorder.
- **Interpersonal difficulty:** Relationship strain, poor communication, avoidance of intimacy, and partner frustration.
- **Performance anxiety:** A preoccupation with sexual performance rather than pleasure, which can perpetuate the disorder.

6 DSM-5 Diagnostic Criteria for Sexual Disorders

The DSM-5 provides a standardized framework for the diagnosis of sexual dysfunctions. The following are the core diagnostic criteria common to these conditions, with specific manifestations detailed for each subtype.

General Diagnostic Main Principles

For a diagnosis of any specific sexual dysfunction, the following general criteria must be met, in addition to the specific symptom criteria for each disorder:

- **Criterion A: Symptom Presence:** A persistent pattern of one or more specified symptoms of sufficient duration (typically a minimum of **6 months**).
- **Criterion B: Clinically Significant Distress:** The symptoms cause clinically significant distress in the individual.
- **Criterion C: Rule-Out Conditions:** The sexual dysfunction is not better explained by a non-sexual mental disorder, severe relationship distress or other significant stressors, or the effects of a substance/medication or another medical condition.

Specific Disorder Criteria

The DSM-5 categorizes sexual dysfunctions based on the phase of the sexual response cycle they disrupt. The key diagnostic features for major categories are below.

1. **Female Sexual Interest/Arousal Disorder**

Must experience at least three of the following symptoms:

- Absent/reduced interest in sexual activity.
- Absent/reduced sexual/erotic thoughts or fantasies.
- No/reduced initiation of sexual activity and unreceptive to partner's attempts.
- Absent/reduced sexual excitement or pleasure during activity (in $\geq$ 75% of encounters).
- Absent/reduced sexual interest/arousal in response to internal or external cues.
- Absent/reduced genital or non-genital sensations during sexual activity (in $\geq$ 75% of encounters).

2. **Erectile Disorder**

Must experience at least one of the following on almost all or all occasions of sexual activity:

- Marked difficulty in obtaining an erection.
- Marked difficulty in maintaining an erection until completion of sexual activity.
- Marked decrease in erectile rigidity.

3. **Female Orgasmic Disorder**

Presence of either of the following symptoms on almost all or all occasions of sexual activity:

- Marked delay, infrequency, or absence of orgasm.
- Markedly reduced intensity of orgasmic sensations.

4. **Delayed Ejaculation**

Presence of either of the following symptoms on almost all or all occasions of partnered sexual activity:

- Marked delay in ejaculation.
- Marked infrequency or absence of ejaculation.

5. **Premature (Early) Ejaculation**

- A persistent or recurrent pattern of ejaculation occurring during partnered sexual activity within approximately **1 min** following vaginal penetration and before the individual wishes it.

This specific duration does not apply to non-vaginal sexual activities.

6. **Genito-Pelvic Pain/Penetration Disorder**

Persistent or Recurrent Difficulties with at Least One of the Following:

- Vaginal penetration during intercourse.
- Marked vulvovaginal or pelvic pain during vaginal penetration or attempted penetration.
- Marked fear or anxiety about vulvovaginal or pelvic pain in anticipation of, during, or as a result of vaginal penetration.
- Marked tensing or tightening of the pelvic floor muscles during attempted vaginal penetration.

Specifiers and Clinical Usefulness

The DSM-5 emphasizes the use of specifiers to create a full clinical picture:

- **Lifelong vs. Acquired:** Whether the disorder has been present since the onset of sexual functioning or developed after a period of normal functioning.
- **Generalized vs. Situational:** Whether the dysfunction occurs in all situations and with all partners, or is limited to specific types of stimulation, situations, or partners.
- **Severity:** Rated as mild, moderate, or severe based on the degree of distress and interpersonal difficulty.

Medical Management of Sexual Disorders

The management of sexual disorders requires a comprehensive, biopsychosocial approach, integrating medical and psychological strategies. Treatment is tailored to the specific diagnosis, underlying etiology, and the individual's or couple's goals. The following outlines the principal components of contemporary medical management.

1. **Pharmacological Management**

Pharmacotherapy is a cornerstone for specific dysfunctions, particularly those with a strong biological component.

For Erectile Disorder:

- **Phosphodiesterase-5 (PDE5) Inhibitors** (e.g., sildenafil, tadalafil, vardenafil) are the first-line treatment. They enhance the effects of nitric oxide, facilitating vasodilation and blood flow to the corpus cavernosum.
- **Second-Line Therapies** include intracavernosal or intraurethral alprostadil injections, which directly induce erection.
- **Testosterone Replacement Therapy** is only indicated in men with clinically confirmed hypogonadism.

For Hypoactive Sexual Desire Disorder (HSDD) in Women:

- **Flibanserin** and **Bremelanotide** are FDA-approved agents that modulate central neurotransmitters to enhance sexual desire.

- **Testosterone Therapy** (off-label in many countries) may be considered for postmenopausal women with HSDD, though its use requires careful risk–benefit assessment.

For Premature (Early) Ejaculation:

- **Selective Serotonin Reuptake Inhibitors (SSRIs)** such as dapoxetine (approved for PE in some countries), paroxetine, and sertraline are used for their side effect of delayed ejaculation.
- **Topical Anesthetics** (e.g., lidocaine/prilocaine cream) can reduce glans sensitivity and delay ejaculation.

For Genito-Pelvic Pain/Penetration Disorder:

- **Topical Lidocaine** applied to the vestibule can help manage localized provoked pain.
- **Botulinum Toxin (Botox) Injections** and **Trigger Point Injections** into the pelvic floor muscles are emerging treatments for refractory vaginismus and pelvic pain.

2. **Hormonal Therapies**

Hormonal imbalances are a key treatable cause of sexual dysfunction.

- **Estrogen Therapy:** For postmenopausal women, low-dose vaginal estrogen (creams, tablets, rings) can dramatically improve genital symptoms of atrophy, such as dryness and pain.
- **Testosterone Therapy:** As noted, it is indicated for men with hypogonadism and used off-label for postmenopausal women. Monitoring of hematocrit and PSA is mandatory.

3. **Device-Based and Mechanical Therapies**

Erectile Disorder:

- **Vacuum Erection Devices** create a passive erection, which is then maintained by a tension ring.
- **Penile Prostheses (implants)** are a third-line, surgical option for men who fail or cannot use other therapies.

Female Sexual Dysfunction:

- **Eros Clitoral Therapy Device** uses gentle suction to increase clitoral blood flow and may improve arousal.
- **Vaginal Dilators** are a fundamental tool in the treatment of vaginismus and genito-pelvic pain, used under the guidance of a physical or occupational therapist.

4. **Psychotherapeutic and Behavioral Interventions**

These are first-line treatments for most sexual disorders and are often used concurrently with medical management.

- **Sensate Focus Therapy:** A structured series of touch exercises for couples to reduce performance anxiety and focus on sensual pleasure.
- **Cognitive-Behavioral Therapy (CBT):** Addresses maladaptive thoughts and beliefs about sex, performance anxiety, and body image issues.
- **Sexual Skills and Communication Training:** Improves interpersonal dynamics and sexual technique.
- **Mindfulness-Based Therapies:** Help individuals focus on present-moment sensations without judgment, reducing anxiety.

5. **Integrative and Collaborative Care Model**

Optimal outcomes are achieved through a multidisciplinary approach.

- **Role of the Physician:** Diagnoses medical contributors, prescribes and manages pharmacotherapy.
- **Role of the Mental Health Professional:** Provides individual or couple's psychotherapy.
- **Role of the Pelvic Floor Physical Therapist:** Essential for treating pain disorders by rehabilitating pelvic floor musculature.
- **Role of the Nurse/Nurse Practitioner:** Crucial in patient education, assessment, supportive counseling, and coordinating care.

7 Nursing Problems and Interventions of Sexual Disorders

Nursing Management for Patients with Sexual Disorders:

The nursing role in managing sexual disorders is integral to a holistic, patient-centered approach. Nurses function as clinicians, educators, advocates, and care coordinators, addressing the multifaceted problems that arise from these conditions (Table 2, Box 2). The following outlines common nursing diagnoses and evidence-based interventions, structured for clinical application.

Table 2 Common nursing problems and associated interventions

Nursing Problem (Nursing Diagnosis)	Defining Characteristics and Etiology	Key Nursing Interventions
1. Deficient Knowledge regarding the disorder, pathophysiology, and treatment options	• Verbalization of questions/ misconceptions • Anxiety about diagnosis and prognosis • Etiology: Lack of exposure to information, complexity of biopsychosocial factors	• Provide Structured Education: Offer clear, evidence-based explanations about the specific sexual disorder, using appropriate language and visual aids • Explain the Biopsychosocial Model: Emphasize the interaction of biological, psychological, and relational factors to reduce self-blame • Discuss Treatment Rationale: Clarify how prescribed medications (e.g., PDE5 inhibitors, SSRIs) and therapies (e.g., sensate focus) work to manage symptoms
2. **Anxiety/Situational Low Self-Esteem** related to perceived sexual failure, altered body image, or fear of partner rejection	• Expressions of shame, embarrassment, or worthlessness • Avoidance of intimacy or sexual situations • Reports of feeling "broken" or "inadequate."	• **Establish a Therapeutic Alliance:** Create a safe, confidential, and non-judgmental environment for discussion • **Utilize Therapeutic Communication:** Employ active listening and open-ended questions to explore feelings and normalize the patient's experience • **Reframe the Narrative:** Assist the patient in separating their self-worth from their sexual performance. Encourage a focus on intimacy and pleasure over performance

(continued)

Table 2 (continued)

Nursing Problem (Nursing Diagnosis)	Defining Characteristics and Etiology	Key Nursing Interventions
3. **Ineffective Sexuality Patterns** related to impairment of sexual function	• Reported difficulties, dissatisfaction, or changes in sexual behavior or function • Conflicts with partner regarding sexuality • Inability to achieve desired sexual expression	• **Facilitate Goal Setting:** Collaborate with the patient/couple to define realistic, intimacy-focused goals rather than performance-based ones • **Introduce Behavioral Techniques:** Educate on and encourage practices such as sensate focus exercises and mindfulness to reduce performance anxiety • **Promote Referral:** Facilitate referral to a certified sex therapist or counselor for specialized, structured therapy
4. **Acute or Chronic Pain** related to genito-pelvic pain/penetration disorder	• Verbal reports of pain during or after intercourse (dyspareunia) • Observed guarding behavior or fear of pelvic examination • Etiology: Muscular hypertonicity, vulvodynia, or vaginal atrophy	• **Conduct a Comprehensive Pain Assessment:** Document location, quality, intensity, and triggers of pain using a standardized scale • **Support Prescribed Regimens:** Educate on the correct use of topical anesthetics, vaginal dilators, or hormonal creams as prescribed • **Collaborate with Physical Therapy:** Reinforce exercises and techniques taught by a pelvic floor physical therapist

(continued)

Table 2 (continued)

Nursing Problem (Nursing Diagnosis)	Defining Characteristics and Etiology	Key Nursing Interventions
5. **Impaired Partner and Family Coping** related to the impact of the sexual disorder on the relationship	• Verbalization of relationship strain by patient or partner • Poor communication, including avoidance of the topic • Expressions of frustration, blame, or resentment	• **Assess Relationship Dynamics:** In a supportive manner, explore the impact of the disorder on both partners • **Facilitate Communication:** Mediate conversations to help partners express needs, fears, and expectations constructively • **Recommend Couples Therapy:** Advocate for and refer to relationship counseling or couples sex therapy to address underlying relational issues
6. **Risk for Ineffective Therapeutic Regimen Management** related to medication side effects, complexity of treatment, or psychological barriers	• Verbalized difficulty adhering to the treatment plan • Failure to attend follow-up appointments • Experience of side effects leading to discontinuation	• **Provide Proactive Education:** Discuss potential side effects of medications and strategies to manage them (e.g., taking PDE5 inhibitors on an empty stomach) • **Simplify the Regimen:** Collaborate with the prescriber to simplify dosing schedules where possible • **Schedule Follow-up:** Proactively schedule follow-up calls or visits to monitor adherence, efficacy, and address emerging concerns

Box 2. Nursing Problems and Interventions for Sexual Disorders

Deficient Knowledge/Sexual Misconception (Dhat Syndrome)

- Provide structured education on the disorder and treatments; explain the biopsychosocial model; discuss medication and therapy rationale.

Anxiety/Low Self-Esteem

- Establish a therapeutic, non-judgmental environment; use therapeutic communication to normalize feelings; reframe focus from performance to intimacy.

Ineffective Sexuality Patterns

- Collaborate on setting intimacy-focused goals; introduce behavioral techniques (e.g., sensate focus); refer to a certified sex therapist.

Acute or Chronic Pain

- Conduct a comprehensive pain assessment; educate on and support the use of prescribed pain management regimens; collaborate with pelvic floor physical therapy.

Impaired Partner Coping

- Assess relationship dynamics; facilitate constructive communication between partners; advocate for and refer to couples therapy.

Risk for Ineffective Therapeutic Regimen Management

- Provide proactive education on side effects and management; simplify treatment regimens collaboratively; schedule proactive follow-up.

8 Preventive Measures for Sexual Disorders

Prevention of sexual disorders is a critical component of comprehensive sexual healthcare, aiming to mitigate risk factors and promote lifelong sexual well-being. Effective prevention operates across a continuum, from averting the onset of dysfunction to managing its long-term consequences. The following strategies are organized within the established framework of primary, secondary, and tertiary prevention.

1. **Primary Prevention**

Primary prevention strategies target the general population and at-risk groups to prevent sexual disorders from developing by addressing underlying risk factors.

Comprehensive Sexual Health Education

- Implementing evidence-based, age-appropriate education that goes beyond reproduction and safety to include information on the anatomy and physiology of sexual response, normal variations in sexual function, and realistic expectations.
- Destigmatizing sexual topics to foster open communication with partners and healthcare providers.

Promotion of Healthy Lifestyle and Behaviors

- **Physical Health:** Encouraging regular physical activity, a balanced diet, maintaining a healthy weight, and adequate sleep, all of which support vascular health and hormonal balance.

- **Substance Use:** Educating on the negative impact of excessive alcohol consumption, recreational drug use, and smoking on sexual function.
- **Stress Management:** Teaching coping mechanisms (e.g., mindfulness, relaxation techniques) to mitigate the effects of chronic stress, a common contributor to sexual dysfunction.

Prevention of Comorbidities

- Promoting the management of cardiovascular risk factors (e.g., hypertension, diabetes, dyslipidemia) through lifestyle and medication adherence to preserve vascular and neurological health crucial for sexual function.

Creating Protective Social Environments

- Addressing sociocultural factors by challenging unrealistic media portrayals of sexuality and promoting body positivity and sexual self-acceptance.

2. Secondary Prevention

Secondary prevention focuses on identifying and treating sexual disorders in their earliest stages to prevent progression and complications.

Routine Screening and Proactive Inquiry:

- Integrating questions about sexual health into routine medical and nursing assessments for all patients, especially those with chronic conditions (e.g., diabetes, cardiovascular disease, depression) or those taking medications known to affect sexual function.
- Utilizing brief validated screening tools to facilitate discussion.

Timely and Accurate Diagnosis:

- Ensuring healthcare providers are trained to recognize the signs and symptoms of sexual disorders and can perform a sensitive, comprehensive assessment to determine the biological, psychological, and relational contributors.

Brief Intervention and Referral:

- Providing initial counseling, education, and normalization upon identification of a problem.
- Facilitating prompt referral to appropriate specialists (e.g., urologists, gynecologists, endocrinologists, mental health professionals, sex therapists) for further evaluation and treatment.

3. **Tertiary Prevention**

Tertiary prevention aims to reduce the long-term impact and complications of an established sexual disorder, improving quality of life and function.

Optimization of Chronic Disease Management:

- Collaborating with patients to manage chronic illnesses that exacerbate sexual dysfunction, ensuring treatment regimens are optimized to minimize negative sexual side effects where possible.

Rehabilitative and Supportive Interventions:

- **Pelvic Floor Rehabilitation:** Specialized physical therapy for individuals with genito-pelvic pain/penetration disorders.
- **Psychotherapy and Counseling:** Providing ongoing individual, couple, or sex therapy to address the psychological distress, relational conflict, and maladaptive patterns that sustain the disorder.
- **Support Groups:** Facilitating access to peer support groups to reduce feelings of isolation and stigma.

Long-Term Adherence and Follow-Up

- Establishing continuous care models with regular follow-ups to monitor treatment efficacy, manage side effects, and adjust interventions as needed to prevent relapse.

This chapter discussed sexual disorders that require an integrated biopsychosocial approach, grounded in modern diagnostic standards (ICD-11/DSM-5) and evidence-based treatment. Effective management combines medical, psychological, and relational strategies. The nurse's multifaceted role in assessment, education, and compassionate care coordination is vital for translating this knowledge into holistic, patient-centered health outcomes.

Take-Home Messages

- Sexual disorders involve persistent disturbances in desire, arousal, orgasm, or pain that cause significant distress or interpersonal difficulty.
- Sexual difficulties are a normal part of the human experience. You are not alone, and effective help is available.
- Openly talking with your partner and your healthcare provider is the first and most powerful step toward improvement.
- Your physical, mental, and relational health are deeply connected to your sexual well-being. A healthy lifestyle supports sexual function.
- Don't wait. Early intervention can prevent problems from worsening and improve your quality of life.

- A team of professionals (doctors, nurses, and therapists) is ready to provide compassionate, non-judgmental, and effective care.
- Preventive strategies focus on sexual health education, early screening, addressing risk factors, and providing ongoing support to reduce chronicity and enhance quality of life.

Sample Short Answer Questions

1. Define sexual dysfunction and write four types.
2. Describe biological risk factors for sexual disorders.

Sample Essay Questions

1. Discuss in detail the ICD-11 classification of sexual disorders with examples.
2. Elaborate nursing diagnosis and management for a couple experiencing sexual dysfunction.
3. Explain the clinical features, medical management, and nursing interventions of erectile dysfunction.

1. Sexual disorder symptoms must typically last for how long for DSM-5 diagnosis?			2. Which of the following is a sexual pain disorder?		
	a)	1 month	F	a)	Erectile Dysfunction
	b)	3 months	T	b)	Dyspareunia
✓	c)	6 months	F	c)	Low libido
	d)	12 months	F	d)	Hypersexuality
			T	e)	Vaginismus

Suggested Reading

American Psychiatric Association. (2013). *Diagnostic and statistical manual of mental disorders* (5th ed.). APA.

Basson, R. (2018). Human sexuality and sexual dysfunction. *The Lancet, 392*(10157), 335–345.

Kaplan, H. S. (2015). *The new sex therapy: Active treatment of sexual dysfunctions.* Routledge.

McCabe, M. P., Sharlip, I. D., & Atalla, E. (2016). Definitions of sexual dysfunctions. *Journal of Sexual Medicine, 13*(3), 291–304.

Nevid, J. S., Rathus, S. A., & Greene, B. (2018). *Abnormal psychology in a changing world.* Pearson.

World Health Organization. (2019). *International classification of diseases, 11th Revision (ICD-11).* WHO.

Varcarolis, E. M. (2022). *Essentials of Psychiatric mental health nursing.* Elsevier.

Chapter 13
Care of Clients with Suicide: Children, Adolescents, Adults, and Elders

S. M. Yasir Arafat and Hasina Akter

Abstract Suicide is a global public health crisis, causing more than 720,000 deaths in a year. It is one of the leading causes of death among youths (15–29 years), and about three-fourths of the deaths occur in low and middle-income countries. Suicide prevention is a neglected area in Bangladesh, where there is a lack of national suicide data, a national suicide prevention strategy, and suicide is considered a criminal offense, justifying the enduring stigma about suicide. In Bangladesh, females die by suicide more compared to males, and hanging and poisoning are the most common methods of attempt. Psychiatric disorder, presence of life events, social isolation, unemployment, sexual abuse, substance misuse, previous suicide attempts, marital discord, and familial disharmony are the common risk factors for suicide attempts. Some dispersed and uncoordinated preventive measures prevail in the country, which seems inadequate. Bangladesh needs good-quality data, decriminalization of suicide attempts considering the mental health grounds, enhanced research and funds, adequate political attention, and collaborative efforts to initiate a national suicide prevention strategy to prevent suicide.

Keywords Suicide · Suicide prevention · Suicide in Bangladesh · Self-harm in Bangladesh · Mental health and suicide · Suicide attempt

1 Concept

Suicide is the act of deliberately killing oneself. It is defined as death caused by self-directed injurious behavior with the intent to die as a result of the behavior. It is intentionally causing one's own death. Nonfatal suicidal thoughts and behaviors with suicidal intent are considered suicidal behavior. They are classified into three

S. M. Y. Arafat (✉)
Department of Psychiatry, Bangladesh Specialized Hospital, Dhaka, Bangladesh
e-mail: arafatdmc62@gmail.com

H. Akter
Department of Graduate Nursing, Bangladesh Medical University, Dhaka, Bangladesh

S. M. Y. Arafat and H. Akter (eds.), *Psychiatric Nursing in Bangladesh*, Mental Health Systems and Policy in Low- and Middle-Income Countries,
https://doi.org/10.1007/978-981-95-8501-4_13

categories: suicidal ideation, suicidal plan, and suicide attempt. Suicide ideation/thought refers to thoughts of engaging in behavior intended to end one's life. Suicide plan refers to the formulation of a specific plan through which one intends to die. Suicide attempt refers to engagement in potentially self-injurious behavior in which there is at least some intent to die. Non-suicidal self-injury (NSSI) is defined as an act involving the direct and deliberate destruction of one's body tissue using methods that are not socially or culturally sanctioned and without the intent to kill oneself. Self-harm behavior without the intention of death. Indicating a clear intent sometimes becomes difficult. An NSSI attempt can be turned into death, whereas a suicidal attempt can be non-fatal due to various reasons. For example, a suicidal poisoning can be saved by identifying quickly and presenting to a hospital; a hanging can be rescued before death, and life can be saved, whereas a cut injury can be so severe that it can cause death. Sometimes, the person loses control during the self-harm attempt, while the intent does not justify the outcome. It is an extremely complex issue affected by various dimensions of life and society. Therefore, understanding the risk factors and protective measures can help in prevention. Caring for clients at risk of suicide requires an understanding of the personal characteristics, risk factors, and available customized interventions, considering age groups, including children, adolescents, adults, and elders.

2 Epidemiology

Rate

Suicide is a global public health crisis that affects individuals of all ages. According to the latest (2025) estimate by the World Health Organization (WHO), more than 720,000 people die by suicide each year. It is one of the leading causes of death among the youths (15–29 years), and about three-fourths of the suicides happen in low and middle-income countries (LMICs). The global rate of suicide was 8.9 per 100,000 people in 2021, varying from less than one to almost 40 deaths per 100,000 people. It is lower in the Muslim-majority countries, with some exceptions on the African continent. Males die more than females (> 2.2 times); the ratio is higher in high-income countries than in LMICs. About 60% of suicides happen before the age of 50 years. The lowest suicide rate was noted in the Eastern Mediterranean region (6.4 per 100,000), and a higher female suicide rate was revealed in the Southeast Asia region.

Bangladesh has no national suicide surveillance or monitoring system; therefore, research studies and organizational reports are the main sources of data on suicidal behaviors, which have revealed various rates. Police data, hospital data, and data from news reports, along with some epidemiological data from selected areas of the country, are revealed as the prime source. There are concerns of under-reporting and misclassification of suicides in the country, as suicide is a criminal offense; there is high stigma, and there is low suicide literacy. The WHO mentioned that the age-standardized rate of suicide in 2021 for both sexes was 2.9/100,000. Research studies found various rates like 7.3, 10.4, 6.5 (hanging and poisoning), 20.6 (in *Jhenaidah*), 30, 14.7, 39.6, and 128.8 per 100,000 population.

Little is known about suicidal behavior among community people and different cohorts, like older adults (geriatrics), and children. A nationwide study among youths (10–24 years) found the prevalence of suicidal ideation, plan, and attempt was 4.7%, 1.5%, and 1.5%, respectively, while the *Global School-based Student Health Survey (GSHS)* data (2014) found the prevalence of suicidal idea, plan, and attempt were 4.2%, 5.4%, and 4.2%, respectively (total 8.9%). One meta-analysis found the prevalence of suicidal thoughts, plans, and attempts was 13%, 8%, and 4% in the last year, respectively. The prevalence of NSSI ranged from 17% (university students) to 40.2% (gays).

Suicide is rare among children. In old age, it is more associated with psychiatric disorders, physical morbidity, and social changes, while it is more associated with emotional events in youths and adults in Bangladesh. Suicidal thoughts usually appear in adolescents. Additionally, NSSI like wrist cutting, benzodiazepine overdose.

Demography

Although more solid data are needed to ascertain, available evidence suggests that females are dying more in Bangladesh than males. In Bangladesh, the majority of the suicide deaths happen before the age of 30. Among the different groups, homemakers and students were revealed as risk groups. NSSI is more common among females, especially female students.

Methods

Hanging and poisoning are the common methods of suicide in Bangladesh (Box 13.1). Other mentionable methods are fall from height, jumping in front of a train, drowning, burning, firearms (rare in Bangladesh), and cutting (rare).

Box 13.1. Methods of Suicide

1. Hanging.
2. Poisoning (overdose and poisons).
3. Fall from height.
4. Jumping in front of train.
5. Multiple medication overdose.

6. Drowning.
7. Burning.
8. Firearms (rare in Bangladesh).
9. Cutting (rare).

Legal Status

Suicide attempt is a punishable criminal offense in Bangladesh. The law mentions, "whoever attempts to commit suicide and does any act towards the act of commission of such offence, shall be punished with simple imprisonment for a term which may extend to one year, or with fine, or with both." Therefore, any unnatural death is supposed to be reported to the police station to arrange the post-mortem examination to identify the manner of death, i.e., suicide, homicide, or accidental death.

Risk Factors

Suicide is an outcome of an extremely complex interaction among multiple factors. It rarely happens due to a single factor or circumstance. Risk factors are still wide, imprecise, and classified in various domains and ways. It can be considered into three categories, i.e., distal factors including early-life adversity, epigenetic changes, genetics, and family history; developmental factors including Personality traits (impulsive aggression, negative affect), substance abuse, and cognitive errors; and proximal factors including adverse life-events, mental illness, acute substance abuse, hopelessness, and behavioral disinhibition. Every stage, there is an interaction among the factors. They can be considered in other ways, i.e., individual factors including past attempt, psychiatric disorders, chronic illness, criminal and legal problem, unemployment or financial loss, problematic personality characteristics, substance abuse, early adverse childhood experience, hopelessness; relationship factors including social isolation, divorce, loss of loved ones, relationship problem with family members, marital discords; community factors including unavailable health care, suicide cluster, violence, and discrimination; and social factors including stigma, literacy, media reporting, and availability of lethal means. In other ways, it can be classified into biological, social, demographic, family, clinical, adverse life events, psychological, environmental factors, community, and media-related factors. Warning signs can guide to measure the risk; however, it is still challenging to predict accurately (Box 13.2).

Box 13.2. Signs of impending suicide attempt (ISPATHWARM)

Suicide Ideation: Having a current suicidal thoughts.
Substance Abuse: Recent start or increase in substance abuse.
Purposelessness: Having no purpose in life.
Anger: Uncontrolled anger.
Trapped: Feeling of being trapped.
Hopelessness: No hope in life.
Withdrawing: from others.
Anxiety: increased anxiety and agitations.
Recklessness: engaging in risky behavior, taking risky decision.
Mood Change: frequent mood changes.

Risk factors for suicide in Bangladesh is under-studied, albeit newer studies are coming out (Box 13.3). There are similarities among the domains; however, there are dissimilarities among the proportions. For example, about 90% of the suicides have at least one psychiatric disorder in Western countries, which was noted at 61% in Bangladesh. Additionally, social factors like relationship issues and adverse life events contribute more to suicide than clinical factors in Bangladesh.

Box 13.3. Major Risk Factor for Suicide in Bangladesh

1. Psychiatric disorders-depression, personality disorder, Substance (Yaba) abuse.
2. Adverse life events-pre-marital affair and marriage, extra-marital affair and sex, pre-marital pregnancy, academic failure, marital discord, familial disharmony.
3. Previous suicide attempt.
4. Sexual abuse.
5. Social isolation.
6. Unemployment.
7. Domestic violence.
8. Academic failure.
9. Demanding behavior.

Various Risk Factors

- Biological factors—reduce serotonin metabolites, changes in levels of different blood, hormone parameters.
- Social factors—Unemployment, social isolation, loan, business loss, low socioeconomic status, stigma.
- Demographic factors—single, low education, living alone, no children, less religiosity.
- Family history—mental illness, suicide, suicide attempt.

- Clinical factors—psychiatric disorder (depression), personality disorders, substance abuse, past self-harm/suicide attempt, chronic illness.
- Adverse life events—Divorce, death of partner, premarital affair, extra-marital relationship.
- Psychological factors—Impulsivity, poor problem-solving skill, adverse childhood events.
- Environmental factors—pollution, income of the country, green environment, climate change, urbanization.
- Community factor—Lack of access to health care, presence of a suicide cluster, community violence, discrimination.
- Media reporting of suicide.

3 Treatment and Interventions

- **Comprehensive Assessment**: Evaluate current crisis, enduring socioeconomic aspects, mental health status, substance abuse, and risk and resilience factors for suicide.
- **Crisis Planning**: Develop a safety plan and crisis intervention strategies considering the current crisis and available support system.
- **Psychotherapy**: Offer individual counseling and talk therapy, consider psychotherpaies based on the situation including cognitive behavioral therapy and dialectical behavior therapy or family therapy focusing on problem-solving and coping strategies.
- **Medication**: Psychiatrists are best suited to decide. Prescribe and monitor psychiatric medications, ensuring compliance and addressing side effects. Ketamine, Buprenorphine, Selective Serotonin Reuptake Inhibitors (anti-depressants), Lithium, and Clozaine have been found useful.
- Strategies to Seek Help:
- Contact a trusted friend, family member, or healthcare provider.
- Call a crisis hotline (Kan Pete Roi/999) or visit the nearest emergency department.
- **Community Resources**: Connect clients with support groups, hotlines, or community mental health services.

4 Nursing Management for Clients at Risk of Suicide

The role of nurses in caring for clients at risk of suicide is crucial and multifaceted. Nurses are often on the front lines of patient care and have the opportunity to identify and intervene in suicide risk early.

5 Assessment

- **Identification of Risk Factors**: Identify risk factors (e.g., past attempts, psychiatric disorders, family history, stressors).
- **Comprehensive Evaluation**: Conduct comprehensive mental health evaluations using validated tools.

6 Crisis Intervention

- **Immediate Safety Planning**: Develop a safety plan (coping strategies, emergency contacts, means restriction).
- **Crisis Management**: Provide immediate support and crisis management to ensure patient safety.

7 Therapeutic Relationships and Communication

- **Building Trust**: Establish trust and open communication to encourage discussion of suicidal thoughts.
- **Active Listening**: Use active listening and non-judgmental dialogue.
- **Education**: Educate clients about mental health, treatment options, and coping strategies.

8 Collaboration

- **Interdisciplinary Teamwork**: Work with an interdisciplinary team (psychiatrists, psychologists, social workers).
- **Family Involvement**: Engage family members in care, providing education and support resources.

9 Monitoring and Documentation

- **Continuous Monitoring**: Continuously assess the client's mental state and safety plan effectiveness.
- **Accurate Documentation**: Maintain accurate documentation of assessments, interventions, and responses.

10 Cultural Competence

- **Cultural Sensitivity**: Respect cultural beliefs influencing mental health views.
- **Tailored Interventions**: Adapt interventions to diverse populations' needs.

11 Community Resources and Referrals

- **Resource Identification**: Connect clients with crisis hotlines, support groups, and outpatient services.
- **Referral to Specialized Services**: Refer to specialized mental health professionals when needed.

12 Self-Care for Nurses

- **Professional Support**: Practice self-care and seek supervision to manage emotional strain.
- **Awareness of Burnout**: Recognize and address burnout and compassion fatigue.

13 Training and Development

- **Training in Suicide Prevention**: Engage in ongoing suicide prevention training.
- **Advocacy**: Advocate for mental health awareness and policy improvements.

14 Suicide Prevention

Suicide prevention is a global challenge. The prevention strategies have been classified into three categories, i.e., universal, selective, and indicated (Box 13.4). Universal prevention strategies aim to include all the community people. It includes means restriction (removal of suicidal methods like rope, poisons, protecting jumping points), sensible media reporting, raising awareness about mental health, substance use disorders and suicide, access to health care, policies to reduce drug abuse, and supportive mental health policies. Selective strategies aim to include measures for vulnerable populations. It includes gatekeeper training to identify the risky individual at community level, and crisis helplines to seek help at distress. Indicated strategies aim to include individuals those have some signs of suicidal behavior. It includes regular follow-up and community support for mental illness, assessment and management of active suicidal behaviors, and assessment and management of mental and substance use disorders. There may be overlaps considering the target population. For example, a crisis helpline can be useful as both selective strategy and indicated strategy. Bangladesh has negligible attention on suicide prevention. There are a few sporadic efforts and suicide prevention initiative (Box 13.5). Crisis helplines are actively working in the domain. The country needs immediate attention on suicide prevention.

Box 13.4. Suicide Prevention Strategies

- Universal strategies targeting all population.
- Means Restriction (removal of suicidal methods like rope, poisons, protecting jumping points).
- Sensible media reporting.
- Raising awareness about mental health, substance use disorders and suicide.
- Access to health care.
- Policies to reduce drug abuse.
- Supportive mental health policies.
- Selective strategies for vulnerable populations.
- Interventions for vulnerable groups.
- Gatekeeper training.
- Crisis helplines.
- Indicated strategies for persons with suicidal behavior.
- Follow-up and community support.
- Assessment and management of suicidal behaviours.

Box 13.5. Suicide Prevention Activities in Bangladesh

A. Clinical services (Suicide Prevention Clinic).

   (i) Bangadesh Medical University-currently ceased.
   (ii) Enam Medical College and Hospital-currently ceased.

B. Crisis help line.

   (i) Kaan Pete Roi.
   (ii) National emergency service-999.

C. NGO.

   (i) SAJIDA Foundation.
   (ii) Society for Voluntary Activities (SOVA).
   (iii) Brighter Tomorrow Foundation (BTF).

D. Means Restrictions.

There were two suicide prevention clinics in Bangladesh. The first one was started in September 2016 at psychiatry out-patient department (OPD) of *Bangladesh Medical University* (former Bangabandhu Sheikh Mujib Medical University). It ran for two hours (11.00 am to 1.00 pm) on Saturday where patients with suicidal thoughts, plans, and attempts were referred. The activities of this clinic have been ceased during the COVID-19 pandemic. The second clinic was started at psychiatry OPD of *Enam Medical College and Hospital* on October 2021 which was ceased in December 2023. The services were available from 8.00 am to 5.00 pm on week days (Saturday to Thursday).

Kaan Pete Roi is the first suicide prevention hotline in Bangladesh, established in 2013, that runs from 3 pm to 3 am (12 hours). The national emergency services line (999) was started in 2017 and it is evidently preventing suicide prevention.

Assessment and management of mental and substance use disorders.

A society called *Society for Suicide Prevention Bangladesh* (SSPB) was initiated in 2016 consisted of psychiatrists with an objective of initiating suicide prevention activities. It has no visible impact. *Brighter Tomorrow Foundation* (BTF) was initiated in 2015 with some yearly awareness-based activities on 10 September (World Suicide Prevention day). *Society for Voluntary Activities* (SOVA) is an NGO worked on suicide prevention since 1999 in *Jhenaidah* district. Later, it stopped its activities on suicide prevention.

Category I pesticide ban.

Take Home Points

- Suicide is a global challenge, where Bangladesh is not an exception.
- There are variations in the socio-demography of suicides between high-income countries and Bangladesh.
- Mental illness and adverse life events are the prominent risk factors for suicide.
- Hanging and poisoning are the leading methods of suicide.
- Psychotrics show promise in managing suicidal behavior.
- Prevention strategies are classified into universal, selective, and indicated measures targeting different populations where overlap may happen.

Psychiatric nurses play vital roles in managing suicidal behavior as an emergency and crisis intervention with participation in comprehensive assessment and therapeutic communication.

Sample Short Questions

1. Define suicide and suicidal behavior.
2. What are the common risk factors and methods of suicide?
3. Mention the signs and symptoms of suicide.

Sample Essay Questions

1. How will you take care of a suicidal patient in the ward?
2. How will you manage a case of suicidal tendency?
3. Explain the preventive strategies of suicide.

Sample Multiple Choice Questions (MCQs) and Sample Best Answers

Which of the following are signs and symptoms of suicide			Which is a sign of potential suicide risk?		
T	a)	Expressing feelings of hopelessness is a warning sign.	a)		Increased social activity
F	b)	Suicidal thoughts are always communicated directly.	b)	✓	Expressing hopelessness
T	c)	Withdrawal from social activities can indicate risk.	c)		Sudden improvement in mood
F	d)	Only adults show signs of suicidal behavior.	d)		Good sleep
T	e)	Sudden mood changes can be a warning sign.			

Suggested Reading

Arafat, S. M. Y., & Khan, M. M. (Eds.). (2023). *Suicide in Bangladesh: Epidemiology, risk factors, and prevention.* Springer Nature. https://doi.org/10.1007/978-981-99-0289-7

Arafat, S. M. Y., & Khan, A. R. (2024). Suicidal behavior in Bangladesh. In S. M. Y. Arafat, M. Rezaeian, & M. M. Khan (Eds.), *Suicidal behavior in Muslim majority countries.* Springer. https://doi.org/10.1007/978-981-97-2519-9_4

Arafat, S. M. Y. (2024). Suicidal behavior and suicide prevention in Bangladesh. In S. M. Y. Arafat (Ed.), *Mental health in Bangladesh.* Springer. https://doi.org/10.1007/978-981-97-0610-5_11

Chapter 14
Emergency Psychiatric Nursing Care

Deblina Roy and S. M. Yasir Arafat

Abstract Psychiatric emergencies require the most crucial nursing care; these conditions demand critical analysis and prompt nursing intervention; therefore, they are very important in the critical pathway of treatment. Emergencies require competency in prompt management, documentation, and reporting. The specified and standard operating procedures (SOPs) for psychiatric emergencies and their knowledge can be a game changer in the care of mentally ill people and are essentially lifesaving. This chapter includes management concepts and the management of psychiatric emergencies like suicidal ideation and behavior, homicidal ideation and behavior, acute psychosis, agitation and mania and focuses on the nursing interventions specifically targeted in managing aggressive behavior, substance use, and drug toxicities and conditions like neuroleptic malignant syndrome. This chapter will help nurses use the nursing process and create their own SOPs and documentation process for effective management of psychiatric emergencies.

Keywords Psychiatric emergencies · Delirium tremens · Acute mania · Psychosis · Nursing care plans of psychiatric emergencies

Emergency psychiatric nursing care plays a vital role in addressing acute mental health crises and providing immediate support and intervention to individuals experiencing acute and severe psychiatric symptoms or suicidal ideation. It is often provided in emergency departments, psychiatric emergency services, or during crisis intervention situations. A psychiatric emergency is a situation where a person exhibits severe psychiatric symptoms that may lead to harm to themselves or others, significantly impair their functioning, or require immediate psychiatric evaluation and treatment.

D. Roy
Faculty of Nursing, KGMU College of Nursing, Lucknow, UP, India

S. M. Y. Arafat (✉)
Department of Psychiatry, Bangladesh Specialized Hospital, Dhaka, Bangladesh
e-mail: arafatdmc62@gmail.com

S. M. Y. Arafat and H. Akter (eds.), *Psychiatric Nursing in Bangladesh*, Mental Health Systems and Policy in Low- and Middle-Income Countries,
https://doi.org/10.1007/978-981-95-8501-4_14

These can include situations involving suicidal ideation, severe agitation, psychosis, substance abuse crises, and acute behavioral disturbances (Boxes 1 and 2).

The primary goal of emergency psychiatric nursing care is to **ensure the safety and stabilization of the patient and others (caregivers and surrounding persons)**, while providing immediate relief from acute symptoms and preventing further harm. This involves several areas.

1. **Assessing the patient's mental and physical health** to identify any immediate risks, such as suicidal or homicidal ideation, aggression, self-harm, or harm to others.
2. **Establishing a therapeutic relationship** to gain the patient's trust and encourage open communication.
3. **Providing a calm and supportive environment** to reduce anxiety and undue alertness.
4. **Implementing interventions** to manage symptoms, such as administering medications or de-escalating aggressive behaviors.
5. **Ensuring a psychiatric evaluation** to develop a plan for ongoing treatment, including referrals to mental health professionals or admission to inpatient care if necessary.
6. **Promoting mental and emotional stability** through appropriate therapeutic interventions, like counseling or supportive care.

Box 1: Common Psychiatric Emergencies

1. **Suicidal Ideation/Behavior**—Self-harm intent or attempts.
2. **Homicidal Ideation/Behavior**—Threats or actions to harm others.
3. **Acute Psychosis**—Severe agitation, hallucinations, delusions.
4. **Acute Mania**—Extreme mood elevation, hyperactivity, risk-taking behavior.
5. **Agitation/Violence**—Risk to self or others, needs de-escalation.
6. **Substance Withdrawal**—Severe symptoms like seizures, delirium tremens.
7. **Severe Depression**—Hopelessness, emotional instability, suicide risk.
8. **Delirium/Acute Confusion**—Sudden disorientation due to medical issues.
9. **Post-Traumatic Stress Disorder (PTSD) Crisis**—Flashbacks, dissociation, extreme distress.
10. **Severe Anxiety/Panic Attacks**—Intense fear, loss of control.

1 Risk Factors for Psychiatric Emergencies

1. **Personal and Family History**

   - Family history of psychiatric disorders (e.g., schizophrenia, bipolar disorder).
   - Prior psychiatric conditions (e.g., depression, anxiety, schizophrenia).

2. **Substance Use and Abuse**
   - Heavy use of drugs (e.g., Yaba, alcohol, cocaine, cannabis) or sudden withdrawal.
3. **Age and Gender**
   - Younger adults, especially males, at risk for aggression or suicide.
   - Older adults are more vulnerable to cognitive disorders or delirium.
4. **Chronic Physical Illness**
   - Chronic diseases (e.g., cancer, diabetes) can trigger psychiatric emergencies.
5. **Recent Stressful Events**
   - Life changes such as divorce, job loss, or bereavement can precipitate crises.
6. **Social Isolation**
   - Lack of support systems or loneliness increases risk of mental health crises.
7. **Lack of Access to Mental Health Care**
   - Limited mental health services contribute to untreated conditions and crises.
8. **History of Trauma or Abuse**
   - Past trauma or abuse increases vulnerability to PTSD and substance abuse.
9. **Impaired Coping Skills**
   - Poor coping mechanisms and low resilience increase susceptibility to crises.

Box 2: Signs/Symptoms of Psychiatric Emergencies

1. **Suicidal Behavior:** Thoughts of self-harm, suicide attempts, or seeking methods for suicide.
2. **Homicidal Ideation:** Thoughts of harming others or violent behavior.
3. **Severe Agitation or Aggression:** Physical agitation, shouting, or aggressive actions.
4. **Psychotic Behavior:** Hallucinations, delusions, or disorientation, losing touch with reality.
5. **Extreme Mood Changes:** Rapid mood shifts, including severe depression or manic episodes with risk-taking behaviors.
6. **Withdrawal Symptoms:** Tremors, sweating, anxiety, or other signs of substance withdrawal.

2 Interventions in Psychiatric Emergencies

1. **Immediate Assessment**
   - Conduct a mental status examination (MSE) to assess the risk of suicide or harm.
   - Gather relevant history, including psychiatric background, current medications, and stressors.
2. **Establish Safety**
   - Ensure a safe environment for both patient and staff, remove harmful objects.
   - Use de-escalation techniques to calm agitated individuals and build rapport.
3. **Crisis Intervention**
   - Use therapeutic communication to encourage patients to express feelings and concerns.
   - Develop a safety plan that includes coping strategies and support networks.
4. **Medication Administration**
   - Administer prescribed medications (e.g., antipsychotics, sedatives, mood stabilizers).
   - Monitor for side effects and patient response.
5. **Involuntary Commitment**
   - If the patient poses a danger to themselves or others and refuses treatment, initiate involuntary commitment as needed, following legal procedures.
6. **Referral to Psychiatric Services**
   - Arrange immediate psychiatric evaluation and treatment.
   - Facilitate inpatient care if required.
7. **Family Involvement**
   - Involve family members when appropriate, offering support and information.
   - Educate families on recognizing signs of psychiatric emergencies and available resources.

Common Psychiatric Emergencies and Their Management

- **Triage and Initial Assessment**
  - **Safety First:** The immediate priority is to ensure the environment is safe for the patient, staff, and other individuals. Remove any potential weapons or harmful objects.
  - **ABCDE Approach:** Even in a psychiatric context, always rule out or address life-threatening medical conditions first.

Airway
Breathing
Circulation
Disability (Neurological status, e.g., Glasgow Coma Scale, check for signs of head trauma)
Exposure (Check for injuries, signs of substance use, etc.)

- **Medical Evaluation:** Assume a medical cause for psychiatric symptoms until proven otherwise, especially in new-onset psychosis, elderly patients, or those with known medical conditions.

Suicidal Ideation and Behavior

Suicide needs immediate intervention and is among one of the most preventable deaths among the population.

- **Clinical Features:**
  - Direct or indirect statements about wanting to die or "ending it all."
  - Formulating a specific plan (method, time, and place).
  - Gathering the means for the plan (e.g., hoarding pills, buying a weapon).
  - Previous suicide attempts (strongest predictor).
  - Feelings of hopelessness, worthlessness, and helplessness.
  - Giving away possessions, writing a will or suicide note.
  - Sudden, unexpected improvement in mood after a period of depression (may indicate the decision to die has brought relief).
- **Medical Management:**
  - **Risk Assessment:** Systematically evaluate the level of risk (low, medium, and high) based on ideation, intent, plan, and protective factors.
  - **Treat Underlying Condition:** Initiate or adjust treatment for underlying depression, psychosis, or anxiety (e.g., SSRIs, antipsychotics). Note that some antidepressants have a delayed onset of action.
  - **Pharmacotherapy for Agitation:** If the patient is agitated, short-term use of benzodiazepines (e.g., Lorazepam) or antipsychotics may be necessary.
  - **Hospitalization:** High-risk patients require immediate inpatient psychiatric hospitalization, often on an involuntary basis if they refuse.
- **Nursing Management:**
  - **Safety:**

    Implement one-to-one observation or place the patient in a room close to the nursing station.
    Create a safe environment by removing sharp objects, belts, shoelaces, and plastic bags.
    Ensure windows are locked and access to high places is restricted.

- **Therapeutic Relationship:**

  Establish rapport and trust. Use a calm, non-judgmental approach.
  Directly ask about suicidal thoughts: "Are you thinking about hurting yourself?" This does not plant the idea.
  Develop a "safety plan" or "no-harm contract" (though its effectiveness is debated, it can be a useful therapeutic tool).

- **Monitoring:**

  Continuously monitor mood, behavior, and statements.
  Observe for "cheeking" of medications (hiding them in the mouth to hoard for an overdose).
  Document observations meticulously, including specific quotes from the patient.

Acute Agitation and Aggression

- **Clinical Features:**
  - Motor restlessness (pacing, fidgeting).
  - Increased voice volume, rapid or pressured speech.
  - Irritability, threatening language, and gestures.
  - Tense posture, clenched fists, intimidating stance.
  - Physical violence toward objects, self, or others.
- **Medical Management:**
  - **Rule Out Medical Causes:** Hypoxia, hypoglycemia, delirium, head injury, and substance intoxication must be excluded.
  - **Chemical Restraint (Rapid Tranquilization):**

    Oral Medications First: If the patient is cooperative enough, offer oral medication (e.g., Asenapine, Risperidone ODT, Olanzapine ODT, Lorazepam).
    Intramuscular (IM) Injections: If oral medication is refused or ineffective. Common combinations include:

      Lorazepam (benzodiazepine).
      Haloperidol (typical antipsychotic). Often given with an anticholinergic like Benztropine to prevent dystonia.

  - **Avoid "Over-sedation":** The goal is to calm the patient, not render them unconscious.
- **Nursing Management:**
  - **De-escalation (Verbal):**

    Maintain a safe distance and keep an open exit path for yourself.
    Use a calm, clear, and non-confrontational tone.

Listen to the patient's grievances and validate their feelings (e.g., "I can see you are very angry right now").
Set clear boundaries and limits in a respectful manner ("I cannot allow you to threaten me, but I am here to help").
Offer choices and solutions (e.g., "Would you like to take some medication to help you feel more in control, or would you prefer to sit in the quiet room?").

- **Team Approach:** Never manage a potentially violent patient alone. A "show of force" (having other staff visible but not confrontational) can be calming.
- **Physical Restraint:**

  Use as a last resort when there is an imminent risk of harm.
  Requires a physician's order and must be implemented by a trained team.
  Monitor vital signs, circulation, and skin integrity continuously.
  Explain the reasons for restraint to the patient.
  Remove restraints as soon as the patient is no longer a danger.

Acute Psychosis

- **Clinical Features:**
  - **Hallucinations:** Sensory perceptions without external stimuli (auditory are most common).
  - **Delusions:** Fixed, false beliefs (e.g., paranoid, grandiose).
  - **Disorganized Thought/Speech:** Loose associations, tangentiality, word salad.
  - **Disorganized Behavior:** Odd mannerisms, poor self-care, catatonia.
  - Impaired reality testing, fear, and perplexity.
- **Medical Management:**

  Medical Workup: Check for infections (UTI), electrolyte imbalances, substance use (urinary drug screen), and neurological conditions (CT/MRI head).
  Pharmacotherapy:

  Antipsychotics: Atypical antipsychotics (e.g., Olanzapine, Risperidone) are first-line due to a better side-effect profile.
  Benzodiazepines: Can be used adjunctively for anxiety and agitation (e.g., Lorazepam).

  Inpatient Admission: Usually required for stabilization, diagnosis, and safety.
- **Nursing Management:**
  - **Safety:** Monitor for command hallucinations (voices telling the patient to harm self or others) and paranoid delusions that may lead to violence.
  - **Reality Orientation:**

    Do not argue with or try to "debunk" the delusion. This will damage rapport.

Gently present reality. Instead of "That's not real," say "I understand that is what you are seeing/hearing, but I am not experiencing that."
Focus on the patient's feelings: "That must be very frightening for you."

- **Therapeutic Environment:**

  Reduce environmental stimuli (e.g., lower lights, reduce noise).
  Use clear, simple, and concise communication.
  Engage the patient in reality-based activities (e.g., simple crafts, listening to music).

Substance-Related Emergencies (Intoxication and Withdrawal)

- **Alcohol Withdrawal/Delirium Tremens (DTs):**
  - **Features:** Tachycardia, hypertension, tremors, sweating, anxiety. Can progress to seizures and DTs (disorientation, severe agitation, visual hallucinations). A medical emergency with high mortality.
  - **Medical Management:**

    Benzodiazepines: First-line treatment (e.g., Diazepam, Lorazepam) administered using a symptom-triggered protocol.
    Supportive Care: IV fluids, Thiamine (to prevent Wernicke-Korsakoff syndrome), electrolyte correction.

  - **Nursing Management:**

    Monitor vital signs and withdrawal symptoms frequently.
    Provide a quiet, well-lit environment.
    Reorient the patient frequently.
    Implement seizure precautions.

- **Opioid Overdose:**
  - **Features:** The classic triad of **pinpoint pupils, respiratory depression, and altered mental status/coma.**
  - **Medical Management:**

    Naloxone: The antidote. Administered IV, IM, or intranasally. Titrate to reverse respiratory depression, not to fully reverse sedation (which can precipitate acute withdrawal).
    Airway Support: Maintain a patent airway; may require supplemental oxygen or mechanical ventilation.

  - **Nursing Management:**

    Monitor respiratory rate, oxygen saturation, and level of consciousness.
    Be aware that naloxone has a shorter half-life than many opioids, so the patient may become re-sedated and require repeat doses.
    Prepare for potential agitation and combativeness as the patient awakens.

Neuroleptic Malignant Syndrome (NMS)

- **Features:** A rare but life-threatening reaction to antipsychotic medication (especially high-potency typicals like Haloperidol).
  - **F**ever (hyperthermia)
  - **E**ncephalopathy (altered mental status)
  - **V**itals unstable (tachycardia, labile BP)
  - **E**levated enzymes (Creatine Kinase—CK)
  - **R**igidity ("lead-pipe" muscle rigidity)
- **Medical Management:**
  - **Discontinue Agent:** Immediately stop the offending antipsychotic.
  - **Supportive Care:** This is the cornerstone. ICU admission, aggressive cooling measures, IV fluid hydration.
  - **Pharmacotherapy:**

    Dantrolene: A muscle relaxant.
    Bromocriptine: A dopamine agonist.
- **Nursing Management:**
  - Monitor vital signs, temperature, and muscle rigidity.
  - Monitor intake/output and for signs of rhabdomyolysis (dark urine).
  - Implement cooling measures (cooling blankets, ice packs).
  - Provide supportive care for immobility (e.g., turning, skin care).

Serotonin Syndrome

- **Features:** Caused by an excess of serotonergic activity (e.g., from combining SSRIs with MAOIs or other serotonergic drugs).
  - **Mental Status Changes:** Agitation, confusion.
  - **Autonomic Instability:** Tachycardia, hypertension, hyperthermia, diaphoresis.
  - **Neuromuscular Hyperactivity:** Tremor, hyperreflexia, myoclonus (especially in lower extremities).
- **Medical Management:**

  Discontinue Agent: Immediately stop all serotonergic medications.
  Supportive Care: IV fluids, cooling. Benzodiazepines for agitation and myoclonus.
  Cyproheptadine: A serotonin antagonist, may be used in severe cases.
- **Nursing Management:**

  Similar to NMS: monitor vitals, temperature, and neuromuscular status.
  Provide a calm, non-stimulating environment.
  Educate the patient about drug-drug interactions upon discharge.

3 Nursing Management of Psychiatric Emergencies

Nursing management of some psychiatric emergencies is mentioned in Tables 1, 2, and 3.

Take Home Messages

- Psychiatric Emergencies need prompt management.
- Nursing care requires expertise.
- Suicidal ideations require extensive monitoring at least every 15 min.
- Always keep sharps and all kinds of self-injurious, risky equipment away from the patient.
- Always keep a track of the vital signs of the patients with psychiatric emergencies.
- Restraints must be monitored hourly for the need and reinforced only under written orders by the treating physician.
- Document the nursing management according to the nursing process.
- Do not skip assessment at any cost.
- Create emergency-specific standard operating procedures and train nurses to carry them out as standing orders.
- Foster clinical co-ordination to minimize risk for injury.
- Practice Aggression management and de-escalation techniques with the team and include them in team-building exercises.
- Prepare a Seizure protocol and reserve few beds in the unit for emergency cases.
- Keep a buffer stock of emergency medications to avoid lag times during emergencies.
- Keep parenteral preparations for the following (Lorazepam, Haloperidol, Promethazine, Flumazenil, Naltrexone, Vit 12, Vit B complex, Inj Thiamine) and set of common IV Fluids like Dextrose Normal Saline, Normal Saline, Ringers Lactate in the unit for administration.
- Document all orders and use 10 rights of medication administration while administering any medication.
- Keep in mind the legal responsibilities and document consent as per institutional policy.

Sample Questions

Sample Short Answer Questions

1. What is a Psychiatric Emergency?
2. Mention the primary goal of emergency psychiatric nursing care.
3. Mention the causes/etiology/risk factors of Psychiatric Emergencies.

Table 1 Nursing management of psychiatric emergencies due to psychiatric disorders

Assessment	Diagnosis	Goal	Planning and Rationale	Evaluation
Patient verbalizes suicidal thoughts, e.g., "I want to die"; appears withdrawn and hopeless	Risk for self-directed violence related to hopelessness as evidenced by suicidal ideation	Patient will remain safe and verbalize at least one reason to live within 24 h	1. Assess suicide risk using standardized tools (e.g., SIDAS)—to determine severity 2. Maintain close observation and restrict access to harmful objects—to ensure safety 3. Establish a no-suicide contract—may reinforce patient commitment to safety 4. Provide emotional support and coordinate admission—enhances patient stability 5. Inform and involve family members—increases surveillance and support	Patient demonstrates reduced suicidal ideation, participates in care plan, and has a visible support system in place

(continued)

Table 1 (continued)

Assessment	Diagnosis	Goal	Planning and Rationale	Evaluation
Patient exhibits agitation, pacing, loud speech, clenched fists	Risk for other-directed violence related to poor impulse control and hallucinations	Patient will demonstrate reduced agitation and not harm self or others during the shift	1. Use verbal de-escalation techniques—to defuse aggression early 2. Maintain safe environment and remove potential weapons—to reduce injury risk 3. Administer prescribed sedatives or antipsychotics—to manage acute symptoms 4. Monitor behavior and ensure backup staff is available—safety precaution 5. Engage in calming activities and therapeutic communication—promotes trust	Patient maintains non-violent behavior, follows redirection, and expresses feelings verbally rather than physically

(continued)

Table 1 (continued)

Assessment	Diagnosis	Goal	Planning and Rationale	Evaluation
Patient reports auditory hallucinations and expresses fear	Disturbed sensory perception related to neurochemical imbalance as evidenced by hallucinations	Patient will identify hallucinations as symptoms and demonstrate reality orientation	1. Avoid arguing about hallucinations—prevents escalation of distrust 2. Use grounding statements and validate emotions—supports reality orientation 3. Reduce environmental stimuli—minimizes sensory overload 4. Encourage participation in structured activities—diverts focus from psychosis 5. Monitor for command hallucinations—essential for risk prevention	Patient acknowledges hallucinations, engages in reality-based interactions, and reports decreased distress

(continued)

Table 1 (continued)

Assessment	Diagnosis	Goal	Planning and Rationale	Evaluation
Patient reports inner restlessness, inability to sit still, and constant pacing after antipsychotic use	Impaired comfort related to extrapyramidal side effects of medication as evidenced by akathisia symptoms	Patient will report decreased restlessness and improved comfort after medication adjustment	1. Assess medication history and onset of symptoms—to confirm drug-induced akathisia 2. Notify physician for medication review or dose adjustment—to reduce side effects 3. Administer prescribed beta-blockers or benzodiazepines—proven relief agents 4. Provide reassurance and calm environment—minimizes distress 5. Educate patient on reporting future side effects—aids early identification	Patient reports improved comfort, reduced pacing, and tolerates treatment regimen

(continued)

Table 1 (continued)

Assessment	Diagnosis	Goal	Planning and Rationale	Evaluation
Patient shows muscle spasms, facial grimacing, and neck stiffness after antipsychotic administration	Impaired physical mobility related to extrapyramidal side effects as evidenced by dystonic reactions	Patient will be free from painful spasms and regain normal movement within 24 h of treatment	1. Recognize and document acute dystonia symptoms—ensures early intervention 2. Administer anticholinergic medications (e.g., Benztropine) as prescribed—relieves dystonia 3. Monitor airway patency if laryngeal muscles are involved—prevents respiratory distress 4. Reassure patient that symptoms are reversible—reduces anxiety 5. Inform physician for long-term medication adjustment—prevents recurrence	Patient experiences relief from spasms, demonstrates normal muscle tone, and resumes normal activities

(continued)

Table 1 (continued)

Assessment	Diagnosis	Goal	Planning and Rationale	Evaluation
Patient presents with fever, muscle rigidity, altered consciousness, and autonomic instability	Hyperthermia related to medication-induced dopamine blockade as evidenced by neuroleptic malignant syndrome	Patient will achieve normothermia and stable vital signs within 48 h of treatment initiation	1. Discontinue antipsychotic medication immediately—eliminates the causative agent 2. Initiate cooling measures and IV hydration—controls fever and supports renal function 3. Administer Dantrolene or Bromocriptine as prescribed—specific pharmacologic treatment 4. Monitor CK levels, fluid balance, and renal output—tracks complication severity 5. Provide ICU-level supportive care—ensures close monitoring of life-threatening condition	Patient maintains normal temperature and vitals, with resolving rigidity and alert mental status

(continued)

Table 1 (continued)

Assessment	Diagnosis	Goal	Planning and Rationale	Evaluation
Patient demonstrates agitation, hyperreflexia, tremors, and elevated temperature after serotonergic drug use	Risk for injury related to neuromuscular hyperactivity and autonomic instability due to serotonin syndrome	Patient will remain free from complications and demonstrate clinical improvement within 24–48 h	1. Discontinue all serotonergic agents—halts symptom progression 2. Monitor vitals and neuromuscular signs regularly—detects worsening or improvement 3. Administer benzodiazepines and Cyproheptadine if ordered—for symptom control 4. Provide calm, low-stimulation environment—reduces agitation 5. Educate patient on medication interactions and overdose risks—prevents recurrence	Patient stabilizes with reduced agitation and hyperreflexia, and avoids further serotonergic exposure

Table 2 Nursing care plan for patients in psychiatric emergencies due to substance use

Assessment	Diagnosis	Goal	Intervention	Evaluation
Patient appears disoriented, unsteady gait, slurred speech, and alcohol odor on breath	Risk for injury related to impaired judgment and motor coordination secondary to alcohol intoxication	Patient will remain injury-free and demonstrate improved sensorium as intoxication resolves	1. Monitor vital signs and level of consciousness—detects deterioration 2. Maintain airway patency and prevent aspiration—ensures breathing and safety 3. Keep patient in low-stimulation, supervised environment—reduces agitation 4. Reorient patient frequently and provide hydration—supports recovery 5. Educate patient on alcohol effects and harm reduction strategies—promotes awareness	Patient regains full orientation, demonstrates stable gait, and avoids injury during care

(continued)

Table 2 (continued)

Assessment	Diagnosis	Goal	Intervention	Evaluation
Patient presents with tremors, anxiety, tachycardia, and sweating; history of recent alcohol cessation	Risk for seizures related to CNS hyperexcitability secondary to alcohol withdrawal	Patient will remain seizure-free and demonstrate reduced withdrawal symptoms within 72 h	1. Assess withdrawal severity using clinical scale—guides medication dosing 2. Administer benzodiazepines as prescribed—prevents seizures 3. Monitor vitals and fluid-electrolyte balance—identifies autonomic instability 4. Provide thiamine and multivitamins—prevents Wernicke's encephalopathy 5. Maintain calm, well-lit environment—reduces confusion and agitation	Patient stabilizes without seizures, shows reduced in the utilized scale score, and tolerates supportive care

(continued)

Table 2 (continued)

Assessment	Diagnosis	Goal	Intervention	Evaluation
Patient appears euphoric, red eyes, slowed reaction time, and dry mouth; recent cannabis use admitted	Disturbed sensory perception related to cannabis intoxication as evidenced by altered time perception and attention	Patient will verbalize understanding of intoxication symptoms and regain normal perception within 24 h	1. Monitor for paranoia or panic reactions—ensures safety 2. Provide reassurance and calm environment—prevents escalation 3. Educate patient on duration of intoxication effects—promotes self-monitoring 4. Ensure hydration and supervision until symptoms resolve—maintains safety 5. Counsel on long-term risks of cannabis use—supports health behavior change	Patient exhibits normalized sensory perception and expresses understanding of substance effects

(continued)

Table 2 (continued)

Assessment	Diagnosis	Goal	Intervention	Evaluation
Patient is restless, euphoric, talks excessively, and shows dilated pupils with tachycardia	Risk for cardiac complications related to CNS stimulation secondary to cocaine intoxication	Patient will maintain stable cardiac status and refrain from self-harm or aggression during care	1. Monitor ECG, vitals, and mental status—detects cardiac or hypertensive crises 2. Provide benzodiazepines for agitation or seizures if needed—reduces stimulation 3. Minimize stimuli and provide safe, supervised space—prevents aggression 4. Administer fluids and oxygen as indicated—supports circulation and metabolism 5. Counsel on risks of repeated stimulant use—educates patient on harm prevention	Patient remains hemodynamically stable, calms appropriately, and avoids complications

Table 3 Nursing care plan: catatonia

Assessment	Diagnosis	Goal	Planning and Rationale	Evaluation
Patient presents with stupor, mutism, waxy flexibility, posturing, and unresponsiveness. No spontaneous movement or verbal output	Impaired physical mobility related to psychomotor retardation as evidenced by immobility and mutism	Patient will demonstrate improved mobility and respond to simple commands within 72 h of intervention	1. Perform frequent physical assessments to monitor circulation, hydration, and respiratory status—prevents complications of immobility 2. Implement passive range of motion exercises—maintains joint flexibility and prevents contractures 3. Maintain skin integrity with regular repositioning—prevents pressure ulcers 4. Provide nutrition and fluids via appropriate route—sustains physiological function 5. Administer prescribed benzodiazepines (e.g., lorazepam) or ECT as ordered—addresses underlying cause 6. Minimize environmental stimuli and speak calmly even if patient is mute—promotes psychological safety	Patient shows reduced rigidity, accepts oral intake, and intermittently follows simple commands. Skin remains intact and vital signs stable

4. What are the signs/symptoms of Psychiatric Emergencies?

Sample Essay Questions

1. As a Psychiatric Nurse, how will you manage a case of Psychiatric Emergencies?

Sample MCQ Questions

1. Which of the following is considered a psychiatric emergency?			Explanation
A	Seasonal affective disorder	(a)	Seasonal affective disorder—Can be managed effectively through planned interventions and is unlikely to escalate into an acute emergency
B	Mild anxiety	(b)	Mild anxiety—Usually manageable with coping strategies and non-emergency interventions
C	Acute psychosis	(c) ✓	Acute psychosis—Correct. Unpredictable course, sudden exacerbation, risk of harm to self or others, requires emergency management
D	Insomnia	(d)	Insomnia—Distressing but not an immediate psychiatric emergency

Suggested Reading

Anderson, E. L., Nordstrom, K., Wilson, M. P., Peltzer-Jones, J. M., Zun, L., Ng, A., et al. (2017). American association for emergency psychiatry task force on medical clearance of adults part I: Introduction, review and evidence-based guidelines. *The Western Journal of Emergency Medicine, 18*(2), 235–242.

Gnanapragasam, A., Paul, D., Sebastian, J., & Sathiyaseelan, M. (2021). Nursing management of patients with psychiatric emergencies. *Indian Journal of Continuing Nursing Education, 22*, 80–92.

Grover, S., & Ghosh, A. (2018). Delirium tremens: Assessment and management. *Journal of Clinical and Experimental Hepatology, 8*(4), 460–470.

Sudarsanan, S., Chaudhury, S., Pawar, A., Salujha, S., & Srivastava, K. (2004). Psychiatric emergencies. *Medical Journal Armed Forces India, 60*(1), 59–62.

Chapter 15
Mental Health Promotion Across the Lifespan

Russell Kabir, Madhini Sivasubramanian, Ali Davod Parsa, and S. M. Yasir Arafat

Abstract Mental health promotion across the lifespan encompasses evidence-based strategies and interventions designed to enhance psychological well-being and prevent mental disorders from infancy through older adulthood. This chapter explores the theoretical foundations of mental health promotion, including Social Cognitive Theory, Empowerment Theory, and the Health Promotion Model. It examines how socio-economic factors impact mental health at different developmental stages and presents tailored interventions for each life phase. The chapter details age-specific strategies ranging from secure attachment development in early childhood to addressing isolation in older adults. Significant barriers to effective mental health promotion are analysed, including stigma, discrimination, access limitations, knowledge gaps, and cultural factors.

Keywords Mental health promotion · Lifespan development · Socio-economic factors · Health promotion theories · Mental health barriers · Stigma reduction · Community interventions

Mental health promotion across the lifespan involves strategies and interventions aimed at enhancing mental well-being and preventing mental health disorders at various stages of life. This comprehensive approach recognizes individuals' unique needs and challenges from infancy through older adulthood (Box 1). Mental health promotion involves actions that improve psychological well-being, prevent mental disorders, and reduce the stigma associated with mental health issues. According to the World Health Organization, mental health promotion is about creating living

R. Kabir · A. D. Parsa
School of Allied Health and Social Care, Anglia Ruskin University, Essex, UK

M. Sivasubramanian
Department of Nursing and Public Health, University of Sunderland, London, UK

S. M. Y. Arafat (✉)
Department of Psychiatry, Bangladesh Specialized Hospital, Dhaka, Bangladesh
e-mail: arafatdmc62@gmail.com

S. M. Y. Arafat and H. Akter (eds.), *Psychiatric Nursing in Bangladesh*, Mental Health Systems and Policy in Low- and Middle-Income Countries,
https://doi.org/10.1007/978-981-95-8501-4_15

conditions and environments that support mental well-being and enable people to adopt and maintain healthy lifestyles. It focuses on strengthening individuals' abilities to manage their emotions, cope with stress, and build resilience, as well as enhancing the social and environmental conditions that support mental health. Mental health promotion is critical across the lifespan, as it fosters emotional resilience, enhances social well-being, and reduces the risk of mental disorders.

Box 1: Role of Mental Health Promotion in Different Stages of Life

1. **Infancy and Childhood**
   - Focus on secure attachments, nurturing environments, and developing coping skills.
   - Programmes like parental education and early childhood interventions are crucial for mental health development.
2. **Adolescence**
   - Promote self-esteem, resilience, and healthy coping mechanisms.
   - School-based programmes, peer support groups, and substance abuse prevention are key strategies.
3. **Adulthood**
   - Stress management, workplace mental health initiatives, and work-life balance support are important.
   - Address mental health within parenting and family life.
4. **Older Adults**
   - Focus on preventing isolation, managing chronic conditions, and promoting cognitive health.
   - Community engagement and support groups are vital in this stage.

1 Theoretical Aspects

Social-Ecological Model: Human development and mental health are influenced by multiple levels of environmental systems, from immediate settings to broad cultural values. This model helps us understand that promoting mental health requires action at all levels—supporting individuals, strengthening families, improving schools, and changing policies—not just treating individual symptoms.

Key Components:

1. **Microsystem:** Immediate environment (family, school, peers)
2. **Mesosystem:** Connections between microsystems (parent–teacher relationships)
3. **Exosystem:** Indirect environments (parent's workplace, community services)
4. **Macrosystem:** Cultural values, laws, customs

5. **Chronosystem:** Changes over time (life transitions, historical events)

Use: Interventions address multiple levels simultaneously. For example, promoting adolescent mental health involves working with the individual, their family, school environment, community resources, and broader social policies.

Health Belief Model: People's health behaviours are determined by their perceptions about health threats and the benefits of taking action. This model guides campaigns that encourage people to recognize mental health problems early and seek help by showing them that support is available and effective.

Key Components:

- **Perceived Susceptibility:** Belief about the likelihood of experiencing a mental health problem
- **Perceived Severity:** Belief about the seriousness of mental health conditions
- **Perceived Benefits:** Belief that acting will reduce the threat
- **Perceived Barriers:** Belief about the costs or obstacles to taking action
- **Cues to Action:** Triggers that prompt health-seeking behaviour
- **Self-Efficacy:** Confidence in one's ability to act

Use: Used to design mental health awareness campaigns and reduce barriers to help-seeking. Addresses stigma by increasing awareness of mental health risks while emphasizing that effective treatments exist.

Theory of Planned Behaviour: Behaviour is determined by intentions, which are influenced by attitudes, subjective norms, and perceived behavioural control. This theory helps create environments where seeking mental health support is seen as normal and acceptable, reducing stigma and encouraging people to take care of their mental well-being.

Key Components:

- **Attitudes:** Personal evaluation of the behaviour (positive/negative)
- **Subjective Norms:** Perceived social pressure to perform or not perform the behaviour
- **Perceived Behavioural Control:** Belief about one's ability to perform the behaviour
- **Behavioural Intention:** Motivation to engage in the behaviour

Use: Helps understand and change mental health-seeking behaviours by addressing attitudes towards mental health services, normalizing help-seeking (social norms), and building confidence in accessing services.

Social Cognitive Theory: Behaviour is influenced by reciprocal interactions between personal factors, environmental influences, and behaviour itself. This theory supports mental health promotion by teaching people healthy coping skills and showing them positive role models who successfully manage their mental well-being.

Key Components:

- **Self-Efficacy:** Belief in one's ability to succeed in specific situations
- **Observational Learning:** Learning by watching others (modelling)
- **Outcome Expectations:** Beliefs about consequences of behaviours
- **Behavioural Capability:** Knowledge and skills to perform a behaviour
- **Reciprocal Determinism:** Continuous interaction between person, behaviour, and environment

Use: Building self-efficacy through mastery experiences, modelling healthy behaviours, and creating supportive environments. Particularly useful for developing mental health literacy and help-seeking behaviours.

Empowerment Theory: Mental health is promoted by increasing individuals' and communities' control over their lives and environments. Focuses on strengths rather than deficits. This approach promotes mental health by giving people and communities more control over their lives and recognizing their existing strengths rather than focusing only on problems.

Key Components:

- **Individual Empowerment:** Personal control, self-efficacy, critical awareness
- **Organizational Empowerment:** Shared leadership, participatory decision-making
- **Community Empowerment:** Collective action, resource mobilization, political influence

Use: Involves individuals in designing and implementing programmes. Recognizes people as experts in their own lives and builds on existing strengths and resources.

Health Promotion Model: Health promotion is motivated by the desire to increase well-being and actualize human potential, not just avoid illness. This model focuses on building positive mental health and well-being, not just preventing mental illness, encouraging people to reach their full potential.

Key Components:

- **Individual Characteristics:** Prior behaviours, personal factors
- **Behaviour-Specific Cognitions:** Perceived benefits, barriers, self-efficacy, interpersonal influences
- **Behavioural Outcome:** Commitment to action and health-promoting behaviour

Use: Designing interventions that enhance motivation for positive mental health behaviours by addressing individual perceptions, building self-efficacy, and creating supportive interpersonal environments.

2 Impact of Socio-Economic Factors on Mental Health Promotion Across the Lifespan

1. **Childhood**
   - **Poverty** can lead to inadequate nutrition, limited educational opportunities, and exposure to stressors like domestic violence, which negatively impact mental development and emotional well-being.
2. **Adolescence**
   - **Socio-economic disparities** may restrict access to extracurricular activities, education, and healthcare, increasing vulnerability to mental health issues such as depression and anxiety.
3. **Adulthood**
   - **Unemployment, job insecurity, and financial stress** are significant contributors to mental health disorders. Additionally, limited access to healthcare services due to financial constraints exacerbates mental health problems.
4. **Older Adults**
   - **Limited income and social support** can result in isolation and contribute to mental health challenges like depression. Financial stress also hinders access to essential healthcare and social services.

3 Key Strategies for Mental Health Promotion Across the Lifespan

1. **Infancy and Early Childhood (0–5 years)**
   - **Focus**: Developing secure attachments and emotional regulation.
   - **Key Strategies**:
     - **Parental Education**: Teach parents the importance of responsive caregiving and nurturing environments to foster secure attachments.
     - **Early Screening**: Implement routine screenings for developmental milestones and mental health concerns, such as anxiety or behavioural issues.
     - **Play-Based Interventions**: Encourage play as a means of expression and social interaction to promote cognitive and emotional development.
2. **Childhood (6–12 years)**
   - **Focus**: Building resilience and social skills.
   - **Key Strategies**:

  - **Social Skills Training**: Provide programmes that teach children how to communicate effectively, resolve conflicts, and build healthy relationships.
  - **School-Based Mental Health Programmes**: Implement mental health education in schools to raise awareness and reduce stigma. Include coping strategies for stress and anxiety.
  - **Physical Activity Promotion**: Encourage physical activity as it is linked to improved mood and cognitive functioning.

3. **Adolescence (13–18 years)**

   - **Focus**: Navigating identity, peer relationships, and emotional challenges.
   - **Key Strategies**:

     - **Mental Health Education**: Provide education about mental health issues, stress management, and healthy coping mechanisms in schools and communities.
     - **Peer Support Programmes**: Establish peer support groups where adolescents can discuss mental health issues and share experiences in a safe environment.
     - **Substance Abuse Prevention**: Implement programmes focused on preventing substance abuse and promoting healthy decision-making.

4. **Young Adulthood (19–30 years)**

   - **Focus**: Transitioning to independence and managing life stressors.
   - **Key Strategies**:

     - **Life Skills Training**: Offer workshops on stress management, financial literacy, and healthy relationships to enhance coping skills.
     - **Access to Mental Health Services**: Increase awareness and accessibility of mental health services, including counselling and therapy.
     - **Promotion of Work-Life Balance**: Encourage healthy work-life balance and stress reduction strategies, particularly for those entering the workforce or pursuing higher education.

5. **Middle Adulthood (31–65 years)**

   - **Focus**: Managing work-life challenges, relationships, and potential life transitions.
   - **Key Strategies**:

     - **Workplace Mental Health Initiatives**: Develop programmes that promote mental health in the workplace, including stress management workshops and employee assistance programmes (EAPs, Box 2).
     - **Support for Caregivers**: Provide resources and support for individuals caring for ageing parents or children with special needs.
     - **Healthy Lifestyle Promotion**: Encourage physical health practices, such as regular exercise and balanced nutrition, which are linked to improved mental health.

6. **Older Adulthood (65 + years)**
   - **Focus**: Addressing isolation, loss, and cognitive decline.
   - **Key Strategies**:
     - **Social Engagement Opportunities**: Create programmes that promote social interaction, such as senior centres, community activities, and volunteer opportunities to reduce loneliness.
     - **Mental Health Screening**: Implement routine mental health screenings for depression, anxiety, and cognitive impairment in older adults.
     - **Education on Ageing**: Provide information about the mental health effects of ageing, including grief and loss, and strategies for coping.
7. **Cross-Cutting Strategies**
   - **Public Awareness Campaigns**: Increase awareness of mental health issues across the lifespan through campaigns that promote understanding and reduce stigma.
   - **Policy Advocacy**: Advocate for policies that support mental health services, funding for community resources, and access to care for all age groups.
   - **Community Partnerships**: Collaborate with schools, healthcare providers, community organizations, and families to create a supportive network for mental health promotion.

4 Preventive Measures

Based on the target populations, preventive measures have been classified as universal for the general population, selective for risky individuals, indicated for persons with some abnormalities (Table 1).

5 Barriers to Mental Health Promotion

Mental health promotion faces numerous obstacles that prevent individuals and communities from accessing services and achieving optimal well-being. Understanding these barriers is essential for developing effective interventions and creating accessible mental health support systems.

Stigma and Discrimination: Stigma remains the most significant barrier to mental health promotion worldwide. Public stigma involves negative societal attitudes towards mental illness, while self-stigma refers to internalized shame that individuals experience. Structural stigma manifests through discriminatory policies and institutional barriers. These forms of stigma delay help-seeking behaviour, reduce treatment adherence, and limit social and employment opportunities.

Table 1 Prevention strategies

Universal prevention strategy	Selected prevention strategy	Indicated prevention strategy
This type of intervention is designed for entire populations regardless of individual risk factors. These strategies aim to promote mental wellness and prevent problems before they start	This type of intervention targets subgroups at higher risk for developing mental health problems due to biological, psychological, or social factors, but who aren't yet showing symptoms	In this type, interventions are provided for individuals showing early signs or symptoms of mental health problems but not meeting full diagnostic criteria for a disorder
Universal prevention strategies are delivered to everyone in a defined population without any need for screening or identification of individual risk factors. This approach focuses on strengthening resilience, enhancing coping skills, and creating supportive environments for all individuals, regardless of their current mental health status or risk profile	Selected prevention strategies focus specifically on subgroups identified as being at elevated risk for developing mental health problems due to biological, psychological, or social factors, though participants aren't yet showing symptoms of mental health conditions. These interventions are more intensive and specialized than universal approaches, recognizing that certain groups face heightened vulnerability	Indicated prevention represents the most intensive level of preventive intervention, targeting individuals who are already showing early signs or symptoms of mental health problems but haven't yet met the full diagnostic criteria for a mental disorder. These strategies require careful screening and assessment processes to identify individuals experiencing subclinical symptoms that suggest emerging mental health concerns
For example, stress management workshops, mindfulness programmes, and work-life balance policies are available to all employees	For example, support groups and psychoeducation for children whose parents have depression, bipolar disorder, or other conditions	For example, specialized counselling for students whose anxiety is beginning to impact academic performance

Access and Systemic Barriers: Geographic barriers significantly limit access to mental health services, particularly in rural and remote areas where professionals and facilities are scarce. Long waiting lists, limited service availability, and a shortage of mental health professionals create substantial delays in receiving care. Financial barriers compound these issues, with high out-of-pocket costs, inadequate insurance coverage, and expensive medications preventing many from seeking help.

Knowledge and Cultural Barriers: Limited mental health literacy prevents individuals from recognizing symptoms and understanding available services. Language barriers, lack of translated materials, and complex healthcare navigation systems create additional obstacles. Cultural factors play a crucial role, with some communities attributing mental illness to supernatural causes or moral weakness.

Personal and Policy Barriers: Personal factors including fear of diagnosis, denial, shame, and previous negative experiences with mental health services prevent individuals from seeking help. At the policy level, fragmented care systems, inadequate insurance coverage, workforce shortages, and limited integration between mental and physical health services create systemic obstacles. These barriers rarely exist in isolation; individuals often face multiple, intersecting barriers simultaneously based on their age, socio-economic status, gender, and cultural background.

Box 2: Importance of Workplace Mental Health Promotion for Adults

1. **Enhances Productivity:** Promoting mental health improves focus, motivation, and engagement, leading to increased workplace productivity.
2. **Reduces Absenteeism:** Addressing mental health issues helps reduce absenteeism by lowering the number of days employees miss due to stress, anxiety, or depression.
3. **Improves Employee Well-being:** A supportive environment enhances overall well-being, reducing stress and preventing burnout.
4. **Lowers Healthcare Costs:** Preventing and managing mental health conditions reduces healthcare expenses related to mental health treatment.
5. **Boosts Workplace Morale:** A culture that supports mental health fosters a positive work environment, increasing employee satisfaction and morale.
6. **Promotes Retention:** Employees are more likely to stay with companies that prioritize mental health, reducing turnover rates and associated costs.

Mental health promotion is essential at every stage of life, from childhood through older age. By using the right strategies and understanding the theories behind them, we can help people build stronger emotions and handle stress better. While there are real barriers like stigma and limited access to services, addressing them at all levels from individuals and families to communities and government policies can make a real difference.

Take Home Message

Mental health promotion requires age-appropriate strategies tailored to each developmental stage, from fostering secure attachments in early childhood to promoting social engagement in older adults.

Socio-economic factors significantly influence mental health outcomes across all life stages, with poverty, unemployment, and limited access to resources creating substantial barriers to well-being.

Theoretical frameworks provide essential guidance for mental health interventions, particularly Social Cognitive Theory for building self-efficacy, Empowerment Theory for strengthening individual and community control, and the Health Promotion Model for motivating positive behaviours.

Stigma remains the most significant barrier to mental health promotion, manifesting as public stigma, self-stigma, and structural discrimination that delays help-seeking and limits access to services.

Effective mental health promotion requires multi-level interventions that combine individual support, organizational initiatives, community partnerships, and policy advocacy to create comprehensive support systems.

Sample Short Answer Questions

1. What is mental health promotion?
2. What are the socio-economic factors that impact mental health promotion across the lifespan?
3. Why is workplace mental health promotion important for adults?

Sample Essay Questions

1. Discuss the role of mental health promotion in different stages of life.
2. Explain the key strategies for mental health promotion across the lifespan
3. Explain some key models of mental health promotion.

Sample Multiple Choice Questions (MCQs) and Best Answer Question

Interventions for Mental Health Promotion include-			What is the primary goal of the therapeutic use of self in nursing?		
T	a)	Mental health education is vital		a)	To solve the patient's problems
F	b)	Clients should discuss feelings	✓	b)	To facilitate the patient's healing process
T	c)	Support systems enhance well-being		c)	To meet the nurse's emotional needs
F	d)	Medication is never used		d)	To provide advice
T	e)	Physical activity improves mental health			

Suggested Reading

Arafat, S. Y. (2017). Mental health promotion or public mental health: The time demanded area. *Journal of Behavioral Health, 6*(1), 1–3. https://doi.org/10.5455/jbh.20161121095655

Bai, A. C. M., Parvin, S., & Kabir, R. (2024). Public mental health in Bangladesh. In S. M. Y. Arafat (Eds.) *Mental health in Bangladesh.* Springer. https://doi.org/10.1007/978-981-97-0610-5_14

Kabir, R., Isigi, S. S., & Candussi, C. (2024). Public mental health and access to mental health services in South Asia. In S. M. Y. Arafat, & S. K. Kar (Eds.), *Access to mental health care in South Asia.* Springer. https://doi.org/10.1007/978-981-99-9153-2_11

Chapter 16
Public and Private Systems of Care for Mental Health, Including Referral System

S. M. Yasir Arafat

Abstract Bangladesh is a densely populated country with about 170 million, where the prevalence of mental disorders is 18.7%, with a treatment gap > 90%. Due to the pattern of disease burden and income category, the mental health system faces various challenges. The mental health system has four components, i.e., public services, private institutions, non-governmental organizations (NGOs), and donor agencies. The *National Institute of Mental Health* and *Pabna Mental Hospital* are the prominent public service providers. This chapter discusses the mental health system, focusing on public, private systems, NGOs, and the referral system in Bangladesh. Additionally, it highlights the enduring challenges and potential ways ahead for mental health services in the country.

Keywords Mental health care · Referral system · Primary care · Secondary care · Tertiary care · NGO · Bangladesh

Bangladesh is one of the densely populated countries in the world, with a population of more than 170 million. It is a lower-middle-income country with a dual burden of diseases. Psychiatric illness is one of the top fifths burdensome problems in the country. The prevalence of psychiatric disorders is 18.7% among adults, and there are about 400 psychiatrists in the country. Bangladesh has a pluralistic health delivery system consisting of public, private, Non-Governmental Organization (NGO), and donor agencies that work together to provide comprehensive mental health services (Fig. 1). Public mental health services are funded and operated by government entities at various levels. It is usually less expensive, subsidized for lower charges, and provides health services for a wider range of people. Public services are crowded with a high workload and an inadequate workforce. It provides psychotropics free of cost in some places. The government services are provided in three levels, i.e.,

S. M. Y. Arafat (✉)
Department of Psychiatry, Bangladesh Specialized Hospital, Dhaka, Bangladesh
e-mail: arafatdmc62@gmail.com

S. M. Y. Arafat and H. Akter (eds.), *Psychiatric Nursing in Bangladesh*, Mental Health Systems and Policy in Low- and Middle-Income Countries,
https://doi.org/10.1007/978-981-95-8501-4_16

Fig. 1 Components of the mental health system in Bangladesh

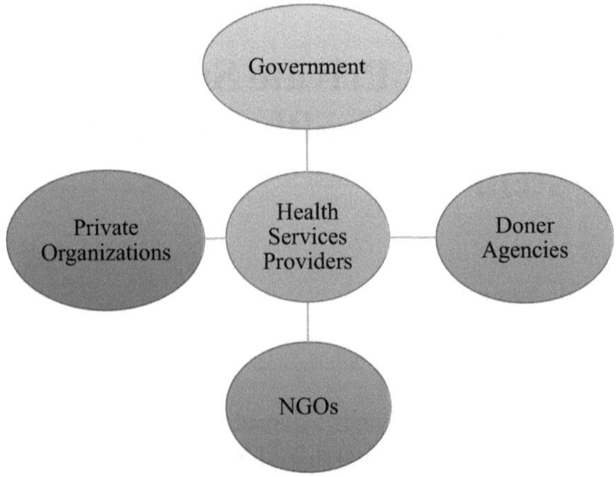

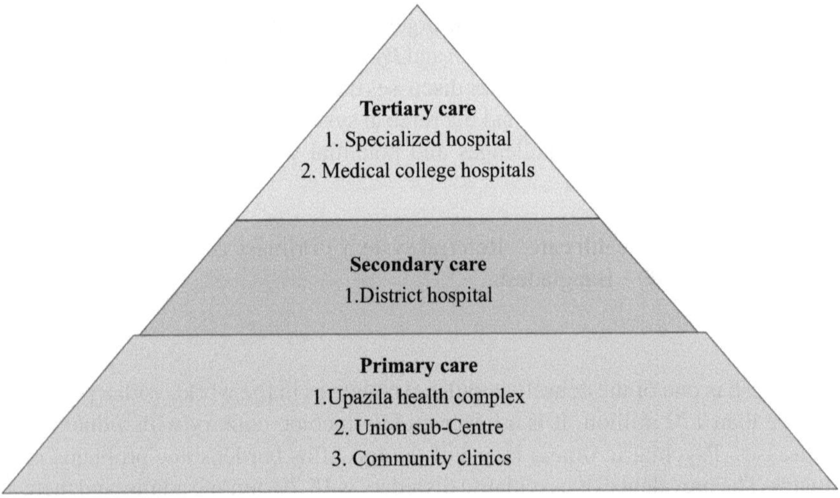

Fig. 2 Level of public services

primary, secondary, and tertiary care (Fig. 2). The historical development of public services is mentioned in Box 1.

Private mental health systems consist of services provided by for-profit organizations, including corporate institutions, private practices, clinics, and hospitals. These services are typically funded through private payments, as out-of-pocket expenses. Generally, private services are well organized.

NGOs play a pivotal role through various activities encompassing education, enhancing service accessibility, fostering collaboration, developing resources, and advocating for policy changes. NGOs in Bangladesh work to **raise awareness and reduce stigma** through **campaigns, workshops, training, and seminars**. Organizations like ***Kaan Pete Roi, SOVA, Moshal Foundation, Achol Foundation, HEAL***

Table 1 Notable NGOs working with vulnerable communities in Bangladesh

SN	Vulnerable group	NGOs
1	Forcibly Displaced Myanmar National (Rohingya)	Action Aid Bangladesh (AAB), Agrajattra, Ain o Salish Kendra (ASK), Bandhu Social Welfare Society (Bandhu), Bangladesh Legal Aid and Services Trust (BLAST), Bangladesh Red Crescent Society (BDRCS), BRAC, Care Bangladesh, Centre for Disability in Development (CDD), Dhaka Ahsania Mission (DAM), Gonosasthaya Kendra (G.K.), International Centre for Diarrheal Disease Research, Bangladesh (ICDDR,B), Jago Foundation, Mukti Coxbazar, Prottyashi, Samaj Kalyan O Unnoyon Shangstha (SKUS), Partners in Health and Development (PHD), Care Bangladesh
2	Climate Change	SAJIDA Foundation, BRAC, Friendship, Coastal Association for Social Transformation Trust (COAST)
3	Indigenous Community	Supporting People and Rebuilding Communities (SPaRC), Manusher Jonno Foundation (MJF), Kapaeeng Foundation
4	LGBTQ Community	Bandhu Social Welfare Society (Bandhu), ICDDR, B, Badhan Hijra Sangha (BHS), Dhaka Ahsania mission (DAM), TransEnd

Bangladesh, BRAC, and SAJIDA Foundation promote mental health education and encourage help-seeking behavior. Despite limited resources, their efforts **gradually foster a more inclusive and accessible mental health system**. They also advocate for stronger mental health policies by addressing service gaps, poor care quality, stigma, and human rights violations. They push for mental health as a basic human right, ensuring accessible care, protection from discrimination, and policy reforms. Their efforts include increasing funding, integrating mental health into primary care, and improving service quality. NGOs in Bangladesh enhance mental health access by establishing clinics, hospitals, and psychosocial support centers like PHWC, and Healing Heart. They employ telemedicine, tele-counseling (e.g., TRIN), and mobile services to reach remote areas. NGOs also train mental health professionals, with 46% working outside the public sector. Their efforts extend to refugees, disaster survivors, and gender-diverse individuals, ensuring inclusive mental health care. Some notable NGOs are mentioned in Table 1.

Box 1. Historical Developmental Milestones of Public Mental Health Services in Bangladesh

1. British period-asylum period
   a. Lunatic asylum at Murli Bazar (now Bakshibazar) in Dhaka in 1815.
   b. It was connected with the central jail.
2. Pakistan period-Hospital period
   a. Establishment of Pabna Mental Hospital in 1957.
   b. Started with 60 inpatients beds.

c. Currently, there are 500 inpatient beds.

3. Bangladesh period

3.1 NIMH.

a. Started in February 1981 at Suhrawardy Hospital as *organization in training in mental health.*

b. In 1988 it was shifted to *Sir Salimullah Medical College* with a 50-bed inpatient facility.

c. Then it was shifted to *Dhaka Medical College Hospital (DMCH).*

d. In 1992, it was started as NIMH at Sher-e-Bangla Nagor with the facility of 100 inpatients beds and outpatient services.

e. It started at the current location in 2001.

f. Currently, there are 400 inpatient beds.

3.2 The Central Drug Addiction Treatment Center (CTC)

a. Established in 1988.

3.3 DMCH

a. Out-patient services were started in 1974.

1 Referral System

Theoretically, community people are expected to attend primary care services, then gradually, they are supposed to be referred to secondary and tertiary care level services. However, practically, the referral system in Bangladesh has no boundaries (Fig. 3). The private sector does not have any restrictions to follow. The public sector does not follow any specific pattern. There is no epidemiological catchment area for any specific mental health services point. The community people can attend any physician, in any sector, and at any level (primary, secondary, or tertiary) in exchange for a consultation fee. Along with the enduring services, there is a strong role of non-medical healers, like religious and traditional healers, in Bangladesh. There is no formal collaboration between the traditional healers and the allopathic treatment system. The potential challenges are mentioned in Table 2. Stepwise nursing measures are mentioned in Box 2 in different levels of health care followed by referral.

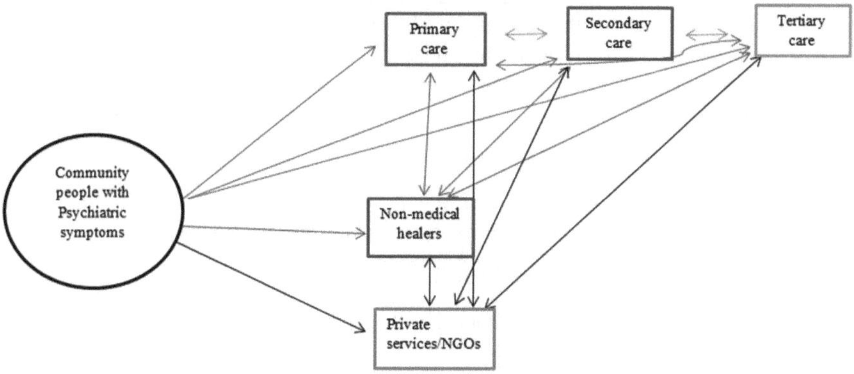

Fig. 3 Referral pattern in Bangladesh

Table 2 Enduring challenges and ways ahead for mental health services in Bangladesh

Enduring challenges	Ways ahead
1. High treatment gap—more than 90% 2. Poor funding and research— < 0.5 of the total health budget, 10 Taka for mental health in a year, only 35 peer-reviewed articles were published on mental health in 2020 3. High stigma 4. Inadequate workforce and inequitable distribution 5. High out-of-pocket expense— > 70% 6. Poor mental health literacy 7. Unregulated help-seeking pattern—no functional referral system and definite epidemiological catchment area 8. Lower-middle-income status and income disparity 9. Non-judicious prescribing (polypharmacy)	1. Augmented budgetary allocation and research 2. Health insurance 3. Country-wide distribution of mental health professionals 4. Expansion of services to the rural level 5. Functioning referral system 6. Additional workforce 7. Provision of psychotropic drugs 8. Awareness creation targeting mental health literacy 9. Good governance 10. Involvement of the clients and their families in the service delivery process 11. Protection of human rights 12. Disaster preparedness 13. Clinical audits

Box 2. Steps of Appropriate Care Through the Referral System

1. **Assess the Patient's Condition**
   - Conduct a thorough mental health assessment (Mental State Examination, risk assessment, psychiatric history).
   - Identify the need for specialized care, hospitalization, or community-based services.
2. **Determine the Appropriate Level of Care**

- Decide whether the patient needs emergency, inpatient, outpatient, or community-based mental health services.
- Consider factors like severity of symptoms, risk of harm, and social support availability.

3. **Provide Education and Counseling**
   - Explain the importance of referral to the patient and family.
   - Address any stigma or concerns about seeking specialized care.
4. **Coordinate with the Referral Facility**
   - Contact the appropriate mental health center, psychiatrist, or rehabilitation facility.
   - Ensure availability of services and confirm acceptance of the referral.
5. **Prepare and Provide Necessary Documentation**
   - Complete a referral form with relevant medical and psychiatric history.
   - Include current treatment plans, medications, and risk factors.
6. **Arrange Safe Transportation if Needed**
   - For emergency cases, arrange for ambulance services or secure transportation.
   - Accompany the patient if required to ensure safe handover.
7. **Ensure Continuity of Care**
   - Follow up with the referred facility to confirm the patient has received care.
   - Maintain communication with the new health care provider.
8. **Support the Patient and Family**
   - Guide them on the next steps, such as appointments, financial support, and medication adherence.
   - Address emotional distress and provide psychosocial support.
9. **Monitor and Follow-Up**
   - Check on the patient's progress after referral.
   - Ensure they are engaging with treatment and receiving adequate care.

Take Home Points

- Bangladesh has a pluralistic health services that consist of public, private, NGO, and donor agencies.
- Public sector is organized into three levels, i.e., primary, secondary, and tertiary care levels.
- Public services are cheap and subsidized while private services are expensive.
- NGOs play a significant role in raising awareness, advocacy, and workforce training.
- Referral system is non-functioning.

- Nurses have roles in referral process among the different levels of mental health services.

Sample Short Answer Questions

1. What are the components of mental health systems in Bangladesh?
2. Write down the referral process in the mental health care system.
3. Mention the key challenges in the mental health care system of Bangladesh.
4. Write down the role of NGOs in the mental health care system in Bangladesh.

Sample Essay Questions

1. Describe the referral system in public mental health care in Bangladesh.
2. Discuss the mental health facilities in the public sector in Bangladesh.
3. List of NGOs working with vulnerable communities in Bangladesh.
4. As a psychiatric nurse, what steps would you take to ensure a patient receives appropriate care through the referral system?

Sample Multiple Choice Questions (MCQs) and Sample Best Answer Questions

Challenges in Mental Health Care-			Which level of health services does a psychiatrist provide?		
T	a)	Limited budget		a)	Primary level
F	b)	High income		b)	Secondary level
T	c)	Stigma	✓	c)	Tertiary care
F	d)	Adequate workforce		d)	None of the above
T	e)	Functional referral system			

Suggested Reading

Arafat, S. M. Y. (2024). Mental Health in Bangladesh: From Bench to Community. *Springer Nature.* https://doi.org/10.1007/978-981-97-0610-5

Arafat, S. M. Y. (2024a). Mental Health Services in Bangladesh. In Arafat, S. M. Y. (Eds.), *Mental Health in Bangladesh.* Springer. https://doi.org/10.1007/978-981-97-0610-5_3

Arafat, S. M. Y., Giasuddin, N. A., & Mazumder, A. H. (2024b). Access to Mental Health Care in Bangladesh—Current Status, Potential Challenges, and Ways Out. In Arafat, S. M. Y., & Kar, S. K. (Eds.), Access to Mental Health Care in South Asia. Springer. https://doi.org/10.1007/978-981-99-9153-2_3

MIX
Papier aus verantwortungsvollen Quellen
Paper from responsible sources
FSC® C105338

If you have any concerns about our products,
you can contact us on
ProductSafety@springernature.com

In case Publisher is established outside the EU,
the EU authorized representative is:
Springer Nature Customer Service Center GmbH
Europaplatz 3, 69115 Heidelberg, Germany

Printed by Libri Plureos GmbH
in Hamburg, Germany